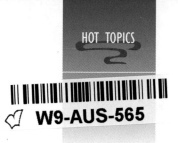
Exercise

Exercise

Manu V. Chakravarthy, MD, PhD
Resident
Department of Medicine
Hospital of the University of Pennsylvania
Philadelphia, Pennsylvania

Frank W. Booth, PhD
Director, Health Activity Center
Professor of Biomedical Sciences and of Medical Pharmacology
   & Physiology
Dalton Cardiovascular Research Institute
University of Missouri
Columbia, Missouri

HANLEY & BELFUS
An Imprint of Elsevier

HANLEY & BELFUS
An Imprint of Elsevier

The Curtis Center
Independence Square West
Philadelphia, Pennsylvania 19106

Note to the reader: Although the information in this book has been carefully reviewed for correctness of dosage and indications, neither the authors nor the publisher can accept any legal responsibility for any errors or omissions that may be made. Neither the publisher nor the authors make any warranty, expressed or implied, with respect to the material contained herein. Before prescribing any drug, the reader must review the manufacturer's current product information (package inserts) for accepted indications, absolute dosage recommendations, and other information pertinent to the safe and effective use of the product described.

Library of Congress Control Number: 2003100246

EXERCISE: HOT TOPICS   ISBN 1-56053-568-7

Printed in the United States

Last digit is the print number: 9 8 7 6 5 4 3 2 1

Contents

Preface

The rise of chronic diseases in the United States and much of the world not only affects economies but also causes the suffering of many innocent victims. In *Exercise Hot Topics,* we explore the epidemiology and the molecular-biological evidence that show how physical activity is a powerful weapon that can be employed in a successful fight against chronic disease.

A major aim of this book is to encourage restoration of physical activity to a level our genes are programmed to expect, i.e., incorporate physical activity into the daily routine and framework of our lives. Another major goal and our sincerest hope is that the information presented here will help alleviate the human suffering inflicted by many chronic health conditions, which have been exacerbated by a real deficiency in regular physical activity in our current society. We present overwhelming and unequivocal evidence documenting the critical role of physical activity as a powerful primary preventive modality against many chronic diseases, including some of the biggest "killers" in our current society: coronary heart disease, type 2 diabetes, a variety of cancers, and obesity. *Currently, to the best of our knowledge, there is no pharmaceutical intervention as potent as physical activity for the primary prevention of such debilitating illnesses.*

Chapters span epidemiology, clinical care, and the potential biological mechanisms by which a sedentary lifestyle produces a myriad of chronic diseases. Thus, all health professionals will come across information in their field of interest, yet will also be able to expand their knowledge base in other areas. Illustrations and graphs have been employed liberally to assist in this endeavor. As this is the first book to integrate primary prevention and physical activity, we hope readers will offer suggestions for improvement.

Readers who will find this book of value include not only physicians (primary care docs, subspecialists, fellows, house officers), but also professionals in other fields of allied health (e.g., nursing, rehabilitation, nutrition, pharmacy, epidemiology, exercise physiology, psychology) as well as medical students and graduate students. Other readers who will benefit are health economists, legislators, corporate officers who must fund their employees' health insurance, actuaries, health policy makers, urban planners, taxpayers, child advocates who work to keep kids out of harm's way, parents who want to keep their kids safe, advocates for physical activity, and policy makers at the National Institutes of Health. We must all achieve an understanding of the molecular basis by which genes that evolved to support physical activity "misfire" in sedentary individuals and lead to chronic disease.

"Scientific research is not itself a science; it is still an art or craft."[1] This statement attests to the fact that exploration of any new field initially is governed by intuition and feelings, rather than precise formulas leading to set guidelines. We believe that physical activity prescription and counseling undertaken to eradicate modern chronic diseases fit in that category, as this is a new art and science, constantly evolving and being refined. As this book is only a first attempt to combine seemingly disparate medical ideas into a unifying concept—that physical activity deficiency contributes to the chronic diseases plaguing our society today—we hope to stimulate new thinking, research, and discussion.

In this sense, this book is not so much a "consensus guideline" to treatment using physical activity as it is a collection of practical tools and strategies to integrate routine physical activity into the fabric of our daily lives. We wish to educate people about the state-of-the-art knowledge regarding physical activity's central role in the pathogenesis of chronic disease and thereby advocate the use of physical activity as one of the prime modalities for the *primary prevention* of chronic disease.

We have not provided all known information for each *in*activity-related disorder, as to do so is beyond the scope of this book. Rather, we have sifted through the overwhelming amount of data that supports the role of physical activity in disease prevention. The reader may wish to pursue further study of these topics.

This work is not the final answer; it is only a first step.

MVC

FWB

REFERENCE

1. George WH. Quoted in Beveridge WIB (ed): The Art of Scientific Investigation (title page). New York, WW Norton & Co., Inc., 1957.

ACKNOWLEDGMENTS

We are infinitely indebted to the American public for supporting all of this research and to the National Institutes of Health for grant support. We thank Kathleen Kolsun, MD, who while at Hanley & Belfus invited us to undertake this enjoyable and educational endeavor. We are grateful to Jacqueline M. Mahon, our present editor at Hanley & Belfus, and to Linda Belfus and William Lamsback, for their patience with our many questions and for insightful suggestions leading to the completion of the manuscript.

We are also deeply indebted to the following individuals for their kindness in patiently reading through all, or parts of this manuscript, thereby making this book better than what it would have been: Espen Spangenburg (multiple chapters); Marybeth Brown (aging chapter); Harold Laughlin (cardiovascular chapter); David Kump (physical activity prescription and counseling chapters); Tom LaFontaine (physical activity, counseling, and promotion chapters); Seshu Ganjam (diabetes and metabolic syndrome chapters); Brian Tseng (pediatrics chapter); Leona Rubin (women's health and aging chapters); Andrew Wheeler (multiple chapters); John Holloszy (for mentioning "exercise deficiency" to us), and Richard Madsen (assistance in estimations of numbers of deaths from *in*activity). We are grateful to the graduate program at the University of Missouri for providing inspiring students.

We are blessed with great mentors, family, and friends, who have constantly showered us with limitless encouragement and support. We are eternally grateful to each of them. In particular, our deepest gratitude to Barbara, Frank, Shalini, Lalitha, and Vijay for their unconditional love and helping us make our dreams a reality.

DEDICATION

We dedicate this book to all people who suffer
from chronic diseases
and to our patients who honored us with a
glimpse into their lives.

SECTION I
Defining the Problem

chapter
1

From Hunting and Gathering To 7–11s and TVs

Let us begin the saga of the modern-day human by revisiting the lives of our Late Paleolithic hunter-gather ancestors ~12,000 years ago. During the Late Paleolithic period (50,000–10,000 B.C.) humans existed as hunter-gatherers, using rudimentary chipped stone tools, and thus are said to have lived in the "old stone age."[1–3] People existing at this time depended almost exclusively on physical activity to forage and hunt for food. Meals generally consisted of wild berries and occasional big game.

Daily physical activity was integral to our ancestors' existence. S. Boyd Eaton, M.D., and Loren Cordain, Ph.D., have written that men hunted 1–4 nonconsecutive days a week, with intervening days of rest, and women gathered food every 2–3 days.[1–3] Lifestyle and feeding patterns were punctuated by periods of feasts (for example, when a hunt was successful) and famine (for example, under drought conditions, or if the hunt was unsuccessful).[1–3] Other physical activities involved tool making, butchering, carrying firewood and water, moving to new campsites, and dancing.

As a result, Late Paleolithic adults were highly physically conditioned, strong, and muscular. The normal lifespan of our ancestors was 20–30 years, and they usually died from common infections, natural calamities, or during a hunt for wild beasts. Thus, in large part, their survival was influenced by the principles of Darwinian natural selection.

With this general background, let us examine in some detail the lives of two hypothetical Late Paleolithic individuals, Mr. A and Mr. B, who have more or less the same active lifestyle. After a long famine period, both Mr. A and B were fortunate in their hunts and encountered a period of rare abundance in food. After the feasting, things changed for the worse: the weather turned dry, and food became very scarce. During this famine, Mr. B died, whereas Mr. A survived.

For the sake of argument, we will transpose these same individuals to

2000 A.D. Such a transposition (from 10,000 B.C. to 2000 A.D.) is reasonable because few, if any, changes in genes or gene sequences occurred in the human genome during these 12,000 years.[1-3] Mr. A is now working as a software professional writing computer programs, and Mr. B is a college professor writing articles and books. Both jobs involve sitting at a computer 12–14 hrs/day. Mr. A and Mr. B eat 3–4 meals/day, and they eat out regularly, which mostly includes fast-food "value-meals." Mr. A's physical activity is walking to his car in the parking lot (which is adjacent to the building he works in) 5 days a week, whereas Mr. B briskly walks back and forth from his home to the college 5 days/week. Their hobbies include watching movies on TV and reading magazines. Mr. A is not only more obese than Mr. B, but he has developed type 2 diabetes at 40 years of age, as well as hypertension and hyperlipidemia. Mr. A died of a myocardial infarction at age 55. Mr. B, also 55 years old, developed none of these conditions, and has now increased his walking to jogging.

The obvious question arises: Why was Mr. A able to survive even after a famine in 10,000 B.C., only to die prematurely in 2000 A.D., whereas his counterpart, Mr. B, died prematurely in 10,000 B.C., but is outliving Mr. A and indeed thriving in 2000 A.D.?

We shall return to our time-traveling friends in Chapter 3, after first considering some basic definitions of terms and concepts.

Suggested Reading

1. Cordain L, Gotshall RW, Eaton SB, Eaton SB 3rd. Physical activity, energy expenditure and fitness: An evolutionary perspective. Int J Sports Med 19: 328–335, 1998.
2. Eaton SB, Konner M, Shostak M. Stone-agers in the fast lane: Chronic degenerative diseases in evolutionary perspective. Am J Med 84: 739–749, 1988.
3. Eaton SB, Cordain L, Lindeberg S. Evolutionary health promotion: A consideration of common counterarguments. Prev Med 34:119–123, 2002.

Definitions

chapter
2

Sedentary

This word is derived from the Latin word *sedentarius,* which means "one who sits." We (the authors) consider sedentary individuals to be those whose physical activity comprises < 30 minutes of moderate-intensity activity each day. Our definition is also based on the recommendation of the Expert Panel of the U.S. Centers for Disease Control and Prevention (CDC) and the American College of Sports Medicine (ACSM): "Every American should accumulate 30 minutes or more of moderate-intensity physical activity on most, preferably all, days of the week . . . adults who engage in moderate-intensity physical activity— i.e., enough to expend 200 calories per day—can expect many of the health benefits described herein . . . One way to meet this standard is to walk 2 miles briskly . . . Most adults do not currently meet the standard described herein. . ."[1] (www.acsm-msse.org).

We propose that a sedentary lifestyle is a level of physical inactivity between no regular physical activity and < 30 min/day of moderate-intensity physical activity, because on a population-health basis, the risk for chronic disease is similar within this range. Since the CDC/ACSM recommendation was made, other investigators have reported that < 30 min/day of moderate-intensity physical activity offered no significant risk reduction for coronary artery disease (CAD), stroke, or type 2 diabetes.[2-4] The same studies showed that > 30 min/day of brisk walking reduced the risk of CAD, stroke, and type 2 diabetes.

Our definition of sedentary therefore includes those who undertake no leisure-time physical activity (28% of U.S. adults) and those who undertake < 30 minutes of physical activity each day (42% of U.S. adults). Thus, by our health threshold definition, ~70% of U.S. adults are sedentary.

Chronic Disease and Chronic Health Condition

Chronic disease is a condition that is slow in progress, long in continuance, and generally incurable. In contrast, acute disease is a condition characterized by a swift onset and short course. For example, the incubation period for a chronic disease, such as type 2 diabetes, is years long, and the afflicted individual typically is unaware of the disease's subclinical existence until clinical testing is initiated. An acute illness, such as a common cold, has an incubation period of merely days, and its clinical course is usually completed within weeks.

Chronic health condition is a general term that includes both chronic diseases and impairments.[5]

Comorbidities

Another category of chronic condition is often referred to as comorbidity—a concomitant but unrelated pathologic or disease process. The term is used in epidemiology to indicate the coexistence of two or more disease processes. A 1996 study showed that one in six children with chronic conditions (17%) had a comorbidity.[5] Compared to children with only one chronic condition, these children were more likely to be limited in their activity, experienced more days spent in bed, and had more absences from school.[5]

Exercise

Exercise is defined by Stedman's *Medical Dictionary* as: "Bodily exertion for the sake of restoring organs and functions to a healthy state or keeping them healthy." Random House Webster's Dictionary defines exercise as: "Bodily or mental exertion, especially for the sake of training or improvement in health." A prominent exercise physiologist (Ed Howley) defines exercise as: planned, structured, and repetitive body movements performed to improve or maintain one or more components of fitness. We believe that exercise has a negative connotation in the minds of many, conjuring endless running on treadmills or performing punishing wind sprints or push-ups to become "fit." Lots of people *like* to exercise, but for those who have a negative image of exercise, we use the term "physical activity."

Physical Activity

Howley defines physical activity as any bodily movement produced by contraction of skeletal muscle that substantially increases energy expenditure.[6] An American Heart Association (AHA) Scientific Statement asserted that emphasis should be placed on play and activities, rather than "exercise."[7]

Leisure-Time Physical Activity—A broad description of physical activities one participates in during free time, based on personal interests and needs. Examples include:

- Children playing instead of watching TV.
- Walking to work instead of using a car (one of the coauthors lives close enough to work that he runs everyday)
- Spending time with kids at the park instead of taking them to watch a sports event

Occupational Physical Activity—Physical labor attached to performing a job.

Daily-Living Physical Activity—Includes both leisure-time and occupational physical activities. This term encourages the substitution of physical activity for mechanical work or sedentary usages of time. For example:

- Climbing stairs instead of waiting impatiently for an elevator
- Walking the dog instead of placing the dog in a fenced enclosure
- Sweeping the driveway instead of using a leaf blower
- Walking to the neighbors instead of driving

Prevention

Prevention refers to the process of intervening or taking steps in advance to stop something from happening.

Primary Prevention—Reduces the incidence of disease or injury by eliminating causative agents. Examples of primary prevention tools are immunizations and seat belts. The AHA defines primary prevention as:

- Educating people about risk factors, lifestyle changes, and the benefits of physical activity to *reduce risk* of chronic diseases
- Identifying and altering risk factors to *prevent* the onset of cardiovascular disease leading to heart attack or stroke

Primary prevention by physical activity involves:

- Educating patients about the risk factors of a sedentary lifestyle
- Identifying sedentary lifestyles and altering the *in*activity to prevent the multiple diseases/disorders associated with the sedentary lifestyle.

Secondary Prevention—Preclinical detection and correction of a disease before clinical symptoms and signs are manifest. Genetic predispositions and/or environmental predispositions need to be determined at the time of history and physical to allow more effective practice of secondary prevention.* Therefore, histories and physical examinations must include:

- Detection of pre-clinical symptoms
  High blood pressure
  High body mass index (BMI)

---

* Interventions that can be accomplished from such detection are explained in Chapters 6, 8, 11.

> Waist circumference
> Pulse for atrial fibrillation
> Fasting total and HDL cholesterol
> Fasting blood glucose
> Hours of TV watched
> Daily physical activity

- Abnormalities detected during the above exam might help identify an individual who is obese or who has one cardiovascular disease (CVD) risk factor. For example, 60% of overweight 5- to 10-year-old children already have one associated CVD risk factor (such as hyperlipidemia, elevated blood pressure, or hyperinsulinemia), and 25% have two or more risk factors.[8]

Tertiary prevention—Reduces complications and morbidities of the established disease state.

Types of Physical Activity

Aerobic—Large muscle groups in dynamic activity such as running, cycling, rowing, etc.

Anaerobic—Very high-intensity exercise conducted well above a person's maximal aerobic capacity. Health benefits are minimal compared to those from other types of physical activity.

Resistance—Loading specific muscle groups by lifting against gravity.

Flexibility—Stretching

Body Mass Index (BMI)

A method to normalize body weight for height. The BMI is obtained by taking a person's weight (in kilograms) and dividing by the square of his or her height (in meters), i.e. kg/m^2. This allows for a classification designated as underweight, normal weight, overweight, or obese (see Table 11-1 in Chapter 11 for additional details).

Suggested Reading

1. Pate RR, Pratt M, Blair SN, et al. Physical activity and public health. A recommendation from the Centers for Disease Control and Prevention and the American College of Sports Medicine. JAMA 273: 402–407, 1995.
2. Hu FB, Sigal RJ, Rich-Edwards JW, et al. Walking compared with vigorous physical activity and risk of type 2 diabetes in women: A prospective study. JAMA 282: 1433–1439, 1999.
3. Hu FB, Stampfer MJ, Colditz GA, et al. Physical activity and risk of stroke in women. JAMA 283: 2961–2967, 2000.
4. Manson JE, Hu FB, Rich-Edwards JW, et al. A prospective study of walking as compared with vigorous exercise in the prevention of coronary heart disease in women. N Engl J Med 341: 650–658, 1999.
5. Hoffman C, Rice D, Sung HY. Persons with chronic conditions. Their prevalence and costs. JAMA 276: 1473–1479, 1996.

6. Howley ET. Type of activity: resistance, aerobic and leisure versus occupational physical activity. Med Sci Sports Exerc 33 (6 Suppl): S364–9, 2001.
7. Williams CL, Hayman LL, Daniels SR, et al. Cardiovascular Health in Childhood: A Statement for Health Professionals From the Committee on Atherosclerosis, Hypertension, and Obesity in the Young (AHOY) of the Council on Cardiovascular Disease in the Young, American Heart Association. Circulation 106: 143–160, 2002.
8. Freedman DS, Dietz WH, Srinivasan SR, Berenson GS. The relation of overweight to cardiovascular risk factors among children and adolescents: The Bogalusa Heart Study. Pediatrics 103 (6):1175–82, 1999.

Genetic Considerations

chapter

3

Returning to our hypothetical Paleolithic individuals, Mr. A and Mr. B, introduced in Chapter 1 . . . one evolutionary-genetic explanation for the dramatic differences noted in the development of chronic diseases, and consequently, in lifespan between Mr. A and Mr. B, is the "thrifty gene." The **thrifty-gene hypothesis,** as originally proposed by Neel,[1] suggested that individuals with thrifty metabolic adaptations convert more of their calories into adipose tissue during periods of feasting. As a consequence, those with the thrifty phenotype are less likely to be randomly eliminated during periods of food shortage because they have stored more food calories as fat due to their "thrifty" metabolic processes (Fig. 3-1).

Possession of thrifty genes by Mr. A in 2000 A.D. still allows him to efficiently store calories as fat. If he goes into a positive caloric balance (i.e., too many calories eaten and too few calories expended in physical activity), then his genes respond by storing fat. As there are no true famines in developed countries in 2000 A.D., and lifestyle in these same societies is increasingly sedentary, the stored calories are rarely expended—and Mr. A becomes more obese (Fig. 3-2).

Figure 3-2 illustrates two key points:

1. If you have thrifty genes that predispose you to store more calories as fat in times of feasting (e.g., around the holidays), you can compensate for the predisposition to store too much fat by engaging in increasing physical activity, by decreasing caloric intake, or both. However, the health benefits of physical activity extend well beyond just preventing obesity, so an individual with thrifty genes who restricted food intake would still need daily physical activity to maintain health.

2. If you do *not* have the thrifty-genes predisposition, you still need physical activity to prevent a net storage of fat. However, if caloric balance is maintained by balancing intake and output (via physical activity), you are likely to remain lean. Daily physical activity is still required, to prevent chronic diseases other than obesity.

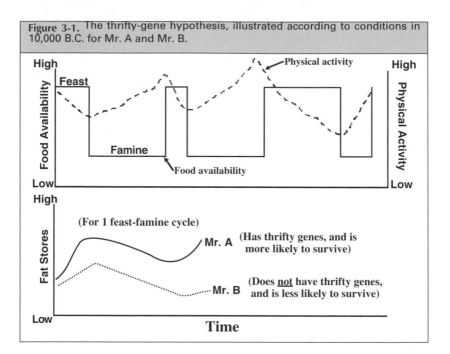

Figure 3-1. The thrifty-gene hypothesis, illustrated according to conditions in 10,000 B.C. for Mr. A and Mr. B.

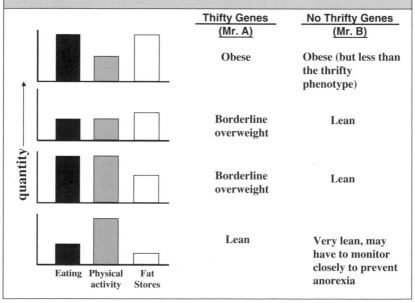

Figure 3-2. Comparison of phenotypes: Mr. A with his thrifty genes that are more efficient at storing fat, and Mr. B who does *not* have the thrifty genes. *Solid black bars* = relative comparisons for caloric intakes (eating); *gray bars* = comparative outputs (physical activity); *solid white bars* = resultant fat stores.

Evolutionary Conservation

Remarkably, while physical activity has decreased and food availability has increased, DNA sequences contained within the human genome have remained essentially unchanged during the last 12,000 years (Fig. 3-3). Neither Mr. A's nor Mr. B's genes that determine basic anatomy and physiology changed significantly over this period. The key difference is that, even though both men experienced a marked increase and consistency in food availability in the last 40–50 years, Mr. A became sedentary, while Mr. B remained moderately physically active.

The way people live in the U.S. has dramatically changed in the last century. The change was likely precipitated by the industrial revolution, but it has taken on a life of its own, leading to an increasingly mechanized society. In addition, over the last 30 years modern society has been dominated by a communications revolution (i.e., TV and computers), and the result has been a loss in leisure-time physical activity. Though food also was abundant and available in the 1950s, it did not translate into an obesity epidemic because the population at that time was not as sedentary as it is now.

The media has popularized the notion that recent gene mutations have produced "obesity genes" in millions of humans. This is fiction. The prevalence of obesity has drastically risen without a change in gene consistency. What *has* changed in recent decades is our daily level of physical activity—there has been a marked reduction. The former Director of the CDC, Jeffrey Koplan, M.D. wrote: "Clearly, genes related to obesity are not responsible for the epidemic of obesity, because the U.S. gene pool did not change significantly between 1991 and 1999."[2] In addition, as noted by Jerrold Olefsky in his recent JAMA article,[3] the prevention of type 2 diabetes requires the identification of the mechanisms whereby the environmental factors of obesity and physical *in*activity convert predisposition to type 2 diabetes into overt clinical disease.

Obesity genes and type 2 diabetes genes are indeed necessary to produce disease. But the genes in and of themselves are not sufficient to produce the current epidemics of obesity and type 2 diabetes. Further, it is our opinion that physicians cannot treat obesity and type 2 diabetes *genes* because no one precisely knows the identity of these genes. However, physicians can certainly identify and treat physical *in*activity! Indeed, a recent National Institutes of Health (NIH)–funded clinical trial found that lifestyle changes, including physical activity, were twice as effective as the best drug in preventing overt type 2 diabetes in prediabetic patients with glucose intolerance!

Most of the current human genome likely evolved in the physically active hunter-gatherer environment from 50,000 B.C. to 10,000 B.C., and remains unchanged to this day. This consequently has led to a dissonance between Stone Age genes and Space Age circumstances, as noted by Eaton et al.[4]

Relative to a timescale of thousands of years, the changes in food availability and physical activity have occurred only recently, while gene structure has remained unchanged from that selected over 10,000 years ago to optimize survival while performing physical activity in famines (Fig. 3-3). The genes of our ancestors were not selected for sedentary existence. In fact, those whose genes only supported sedentary living were likely eliminated from the gene pool.

Physical Activity Required For Expression of Genome

We speculate that "physical activity genes" require physical activity to express appropriate proteins. Thus, when an individual does not experience daily physical activity (i.e., has a **physical activity deficiency**), the genes "mis-express" their protein products, leading ultimately to potential pathologic states. One example of a physical activity gene that is mis-expressed with a sedentary lifestyle is the GLUT4 gene. GLUT4 protein is decreased within days of becoming sedentary. GLUT4, as the rate-limiting protein to remove glucose from blood, fails to move glucose into skeletal muscle when skeletal muscle is not used. The lack of GLUT4 protein is a major contributor to whole-body insulin resistance that occurs within *days* of becoming sedentary and is one initiator of the type 2 diabetic epidemic.

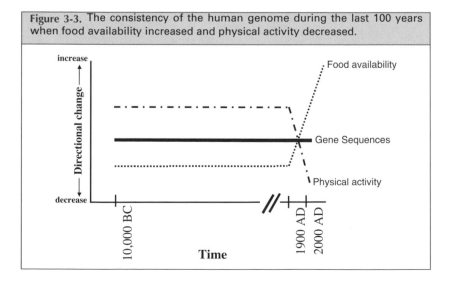

Figure 3-3. The consistency of the human genome during the last 100 years when food availability increased and physical activity decreased.

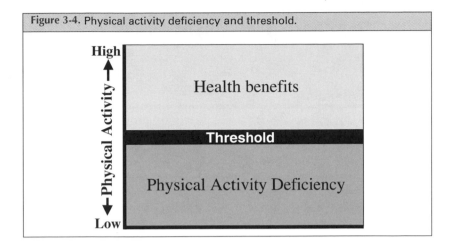

Figure 3-4. Physical activity deficiency and threshold.

A **physical activity threshold** is required for proper expression of physical activity genes, and thus for health benefits to occur. Falling below this threshold results in physical activity deficiency (PAD; Fig. 3-4).

PAD has an evolutionary basis in that physical activity has been programmed into human genomes since the late Paleolithic era (10,000 B.C.). Therefore, our genomes expect and demand a certain threshold of physical activity for the normal functioning of our genes. (See Chapter 25 for further development of this concept.) Current sedentary lifestyles lead to discordance in gene-environment interactions, and thus predispose the

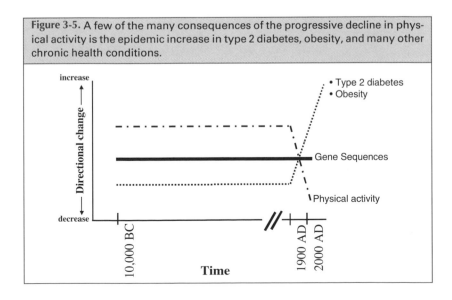

Figure 3-5. A few of the many consequences of the progressive decline in physical activity is the epidemic increase in type 2 diabetes, obesity, and many other chronic health conditions.

programmed genome to misexpress its genes in multiple organ systems, ultimately resulting in many of the modern chronic health conditions. (See Chapters 13–24 for biological evidence of this theory.)

Suggested Reading

1.   Neel JV. Diabetes mellitus: A "thrifty" genotype rendered detrimental by "progress." Am. J Hum Genet 14: 353–362, 1962.
2.   Mokdad AH, Bowman BA, Ford ES, et al. The continuing epidemics of obesity and diabetes in the United States. JAMA 286: 1195–1200, 2001.
3.   Olefsky JM. Prospects for research in diabetes mellitus. JAMA 285: 628–632, 2001.
4.   Eaton SB, Cordain L, Lindeberg S. Evolutionary health promotion: A consideration of common counterarguments. Prev Med 34:119–123, 2002.

Physical Activity Deficiency

chapter

4

We believe that physical activity deficiency (PAD) = disease/disorders. If you are skeptical of this statement, we hope that by the end of this book you begin to agree that a physically inactive state is the harbinger of unhealthy conditions and is a prime contributing cause to the epidemic increase in diabetes, obesity, and many of the other chronic health conditions (CHCs). Furthermore, it is our aim to encourage the use of physical activity as a primary prevention modality to prevent CHCs in the first place, and more importantly, to enhance patients' overall well-being and quality of life.

The world's population at large is not getting healthier: it is getting older and unhealthier by the day, particularly in the United States. According to the CDC, obesity and diabetes are now epidemics. It is predicted that there will be 300 million cases of type 2 diabetes in the world by the year 2025.[13] As will be shown in this chapter, many other CHCs are now reaching epidemic proportions. We believe that, just as other deficiencies can cause disease (e.g., lack of iodine leading to goiter, and then to hypothyroidism; inadequate vitamin C leading to scurvy), our current population's deficiency in physical activity directly contributes to this burgeoning of CHCs.

Scope of the Physical Activity Deficiency Problem

An Independent Risk Factor

Sedentary behavior is an independent risk factor for increased incidence and progression of chronic health conditions (CHCs; Table 4–1). It is also an independent risk factor for increased mortality from CHCs. In fact, the majority of U.S. deaths are now from CHCs.
- 7 of 10 deaths (1.7 million of 2.4 million deaths) in the U.S. in 1999 were due to CHCs (Table 4–2).
- U.S. data 1987–1990 show that there were 1.6 million deaths from

| TABLE 4–1. Effect of Physical Activity Deficiency On Some Chronic Health Conditions ||
Increases Incidence of These Conditions	Worsens/Increases Progression of These Conditions
Coronary artery disease (angina/MI)	Chemotherapy
Arthritis	Chronic back pain
Arrhythmias	Debilitating illnesses
Colon cancer	Disease cachexia
Congestive heart failure	Falls resulting in broken hips
Depression	Physical frailty
Gallstone disease	Spinal cord injury
Gastrointestinal reflux disease	Stroke
High blood triglycerides	Vertebral/femoral fractures
High blood cholesterol	
Hypertension	
Reduced cognitive function	
Low blood HDL	
Obesity	
Osteoporosis	
Pancreatic cancer	
Peripheral vascular disease	
Physical frailty	
Premature mortality	
Sleep apnea	
Stroke	
Type-2 diabetes	

chronic diseases, which represented 24.3 million years lost, with an average of 14.8 years lost per death.[1]

- No regular exercise accounted for 256,686 deaths from CHCs according to 1986 CDC data, and these deaths constituted ~12% of the total 2.1 million deaths that occurred in 1986[2]:

| TABLE 4–2. Number of U.S. Deaths From CHCs in 1999 ||
Disease	Deaths
Heart	725,192
Cancer	549,838
Cerebrovascular diseases	167,366
Chronic lower respiratory diseases	124,181
Diabetes	68,730
Alzheimer's disease	44,536
Data is from the National Vital Statistics Report, U.S. Centers for Disease Control	

205,254 deaths from coronary heart disease (35% of these deaths)
43,063 deaths from stroke (29% of these deaths)
8369 deaths from colon cancer (15% of these deaths)
Deaths from type 2 diabetes were not determined in this study.

- As the U.S. population grew 17% from 1986 to 2000, the adjusted premature number of deaths from no regular exercise is 300,000 (excluding diabetes, as the 1986 report did not include it). Diabetes is included in the next estimate.

Sedentary Lifestyle and Premature Death

Sedentary lifestyle accounted for 334,144 premature deaths in the U.S. from CHCs, according to our estimates (Table 4–3), which are based on numbers of deaths reported on the American Heart Association, American Diabetes Association, and American Cancer Society web sites. Percentage reductions of deaths were taken from the percentage of prevalence when physically inactive populations were compared to moderately physically active populations in the literature (see Chapters 13–15).

The number of deaths from sedentary living is three times greater than that from microbial agents and also exceeds all deaths from firearms, illicit usage of drugs, sexually transmitted diseases, and motor vehicle accidents.[12] The number of deaths due to physical *in*activity (334,000

TABLE 4–3. Benefits of Moderate Physical Activity*					
	Chronic Health Condition				
	CHD, Stroke	**Diabetes**	**Colon Cancer**	**Pancreatic Cancer**	**Melanoma**
Total deaths	687,025	198,140	48,100	29,700	9600
No. of persons saved from premature death by physical activity+	68,937	19,596	8488	2937	949
No. of sedentary persons that *could* be saved from premature death by physical activity#	160,852	45,725	19,806	6854	2215
No. of persons saved if 100% of population were physically active	229,789	65,321	28,294	9791	3164
Of total U.S. deaths, portion saved by physical activity	30%	30%	50%	30%	30%

* Moderate physical activity = more than 30 min/day, 5–7 days/wk
+ 30% of population is physically active
# 70% of population is sedentary

annual premature deaths in the U.S.) trails tobacco (430,000), but exceeds obesity (300,000). Thus, a major cause of death in the U.S. is sedentary living. Physical *in*activity is one of the top two causes of all-cause mortality in the U.S. today, and directly contributes to the current third-highest death rate in the country, which is obesity.

In the last 100 years, the leading causes of death have dramatically shifted from the scourge of infectious diseases (in 1900), to cardiovascular diseases, obesity, and type 2 diabetes mellitus (in 2000)—all of which are directly associated with sedentary living. In essence, physical inactivity constitutes the new scourge for humanity. Some site-specific cancers, such as colon cancer, are also associated with sedentary lifestyle.

Sedentary Death Syndrome

We have coined the phrase "sedentary death syndrome" (SeDS) to categorize the emerging entity of sedentary lifestyle–mediated disorders that ultimately result in increased mortality. We believe this term is appropriate, considering that the word "syndrome" is from the Greek word *syndromé*, which means "running together." Currently, a syndrome is defined as "a group of symptoms that together are characteristic of a specific disorder, disease, or the like" (Random House, 1997), where disease is defined as "an interruption, cessation, or disorder of body function, system, or organ" (Stedman's Medical Dictionary, 2000). The symptom set that characterizes SeDS includes weak skeletal muscles, bone density loss, hyperglycemia, glucosuria, low serum HDL, obesity, lowered physical endurance, and resting tachycardia.

Approximately 14% of deaths in the U.S. are premature due to SeDS. We believe that 14% of a causal factor deserves a name, to focus physicians on the critical importance of physical *in*activity as a direct contributor to the epidemic rise in CHCs.

Epidemiological Considerations

Chronic health disorders are the most common type of conditions seen in the primary care setting. The natural history of chronic health conditions (CHCs) usually spans many decades and includes transient periods of acute exacerbation or alleviation. Unless screened, the affected patient generally is unaware of the problem and may live with the disorder much of his or her life, until end organ damage occurs.

Approximately 90 million U.S. inhabitants had one or more CHCs in 1987 (88.5 million of those were in non-institutionalized settings, and 1.5 million persons lived in nursing or personal care homes), and 32.2 million of these persons suffered activity limitations as a result.[1] Rates of chronic conditions varied with age and were highest among the elderly. The following had at least one chronic condition:

> 88% of the elderly (>65 yrs)
> 68% of 45–64 year olds
> 35% of 18–44 year olds
> 25% of those 18 years old and younger.

However, due to the absolute size of each of these age groups, adults 18 to 64 years old accounted for 60% of all *non-institutionalized* persons with chronic conditions. This age group (the "baby boomers") is gradually moving into the > 65-years-old group, so the number of CHCs will continue to rise unless primary prevention is practiced more vigorously. We contend that eradication of physical inactivity will reduce the number of CHCs.

Vital Statistics on the Prevalence of Specific CHCs

Coronary Heart Disease

- Number one cause of death in the United States in the 20th century for every year but one (1918)
- Primary cause of 949,619 deaths (41% of all deaths) in 1998 and was the primary or contributing cause of 1.4 million deaths (60% of all deaths)
- Claims more lives each year than the next seven prevalent causes of death combined, and the number of people dying from diseases of the heart has risen by 37% (200,000 additional yearly deaths) from 1950 to 1996, while the total U.S. population increased by 43%.
- Although annual death rates from cardiovascular disease have just recently begun to decline (21.3% from 1986 to 1996), the absolute number of cardiovascular deaths declined only 2% in the same 10-yr period due to an increase in the U.S. population.

Type 2 Diabetes Mellitus

- The CDC now calls the increase in type 2 diabetes an epidemic.[5]
- A five-fold increase in prevalence of type 2 diabetes occurred between 1958 and 1993.
- More than 400,000 people with diabetes die each year, half of them just because of diabetes (American Diabetes Association, 2001). The number of deaths from diabetes is sure to rise (see below). Older textbooks of internal medicine assert that type 2 diabetes is a disease rarely seen in persons under the age of 40. The 2001 edition of Harrison's Principles of Internal Medicine now acknowledges that adult-onset diabetes is clinically present in overweight adolescents.

- Onset of type 2 diabetes at an early age makes these individuals susceptible to diabetes-associated comorbidities, such as blindness, end-stage renal disease, amputations, heart disease, and strokes, much earlier in life.
- A recent publication by Boyle et al[3] predicts that the number of Americans with diagnosed diabetes is projected to increase 165%, from 11 million in 2000 (prevalence of 4%) to 29 million in 2050 (prevalence of 7.2%). Further—
  1. The largest percent increase in diagnosed diabetes will be among those aged 75 years (+271% in women and +437% in men).
  2. The fastest growing ethnic group with diagnosed diabetes is expected to be black males (+ 363% from 2000 to 2050), then black females (+217%), white males (+148%), and white females (+107%).
  3. Of the projected 18 million increase in the number of cases of diabetes in 2050, 37% are due to changes in demographic composition, 27% are due to population growth, and 36% are due to increasing prevalence rates.

Overweight/Obesity

Children/Adolescents (for more details, please refer to Chapter 5)
- Like adults, the number of overweight children and adolescents in the U.S. also increased 1960–1962 and 1988–1994, with a similar acceleration in the rate of increase during the 1980s.[4]
- During 1988–1994, approximately 11% of U.S. children and adolescents were reportedly overweight. Moreover, the 90% increase in proportion of obese persons in the 18- to 29-yr-old age group from 1991 (with a 7.1% prevalent of obesity) to 2000 (with a 13.5% prevalence)[5] indicates that those shocking statistics in children are now repeating in the young adult population.
- The obesity epidemic is like the type 2 diabetes epidemic in that its advance is not just a function of more individuals reaching middle age. Rather, these statistics indicate that these are problems originating in childhood and adolescence.

Adults

Overweight (BMI = 25–29.9 kg/m²)
- Percentage increased to 56.4% in 2000, compared with 45% in 1991.[5]
- The average rate of rise in obesity in the last 10 years accelerated to 6.1% per year, compared to a 2.2% per year increase 1960–1994.[4]

Obesity (BMI = 30–39.9 kg/m²)

- The CDC now calls the increase in obesity an epidemic.[5]
- Obesity was estimated to annually account for 280,000–325,000 deaths in the U.S. using 1991 statistics,[6] and this number is likely growing.
- The CDC documented the prevalence of obesity in 2000 as being 19.8% among U.S. adults, reflecting a 61% increase since 1991.[5]
- A study of the obesity epidemic reports that a total of 38.8 million U.S. adults were obese (19.6 million men and 19.2 million women) in the year 2000.[5]

Morbid obesity (BMI > 40 kg/m²)
- The CDC documented the prevalence of morbid obesity in 2000 as being 2.1%, compared to 0.9% in 1991.[5]

Obesity-Related Disorders

- Obesity is a comorbidity of some of the most prevalent diseases in modern civilization.
- The prevalence of comorbidities rises with increasing BMI.
- BMIs > 35 kg/m² are associated with a 93-fold and 42-fold increased risk of type 2 diabetes in women and men, respectively.[7]
- The risk of coronary heart disease is increased 86% by a 20% rise in body weight in men; this risk is increased 3.6-fold in obese women.[8]
- A higher prevalence of diseases such as hypertension, osteoarthritis, and gallbladder disease is also associated with increasing obesity.[7,8]

Aging Population

- The average age of the U.S. population is getting older, and will continue to do so.
- Currently, 3.5 million U.S. citizens are ≥ 85 years old.
- There will be a substantial increase in the relative size of the elderly population after the year 2011, when the oldest members of the baby-boom cohort (people born in 1946) reach the age of 65.
- The U.S. Census Bureau projects that, by the year 2040, there will be at least 8–13 million Americans ≥ 85 years old.[9]
- 25% of all women and 15% of all men ≥ 84 years old lived in nursing homes in the 1990s.[9]
- Most chronic diseases are also considered age-related diseases, since they clinically manifest themselves to a greater degree later in life.[7]
- It is logical to expect the prevalence of modern chronic disorders to rise in future years due to the progressive aging of the U.S. population and the increasing prevalence of CHCs in younger age groups.
- Increased healthcare costs are inevitable due to the rise in CHCs,

unless we soon find a way to implement better preventive measures against the rampant progression of chronic diseases.

Physical Inactivity Is Costly

Economic Costs of Sedentary Lifestyle

Based on recent reports,[1] CHCs in 1987:

- Accounted for 76% of the direct medical care costs in the U.S. while affecting only 46% of persons with medical problems
- Cost $272.2 billion in health services and supplies for non-institutionalized persons
- Averaged $3074 in annual healthcare costs per person, compared with $817 for persons with only acute conditions. Persons with > 1 chronic condition spent $4672 per year, compared with $1829 for persons with only 1 chronic condition.
- Amounted to $161.3 billion or an average of $98,304 per death (indirect costs)
- Accounted for disproportionately greater utilization and, hence, cost of healthcare resources, both services and supplies. Almost 96% of homecare visits, 83% of prescription drug use, 66% of physician visits, and 55% of emergency department visits were made by persons with CHCs, and they represented 69% of hospital admissions, requiring longer hospital stays (7.8 days) compared to persons without chronic health conditions (4.3 days).
- The direct and indirect costs of sedentary lifestyle were reported to be in excess of $150 billion (cost in 2000 dollars for 1987 incidences).[10]
- The proportion of direct medical costs associated with physical inactivity in U.S. adults with arthritis was $1250/patient (2000 year dollars), which is about 12.4% of direct costs for this disorder, or about $8 billion/yr.[11]

Morbidity & Mortality Costs of Sedentary Lifestyle

- Sedentary lifestyle accounted for 334,144 deaths from various CHCs, according to our estimates of the most recent data and literature.
- CHCs ultimately diminish patients' overall well-being and quality of life.

Key Points: Physical Activity Deficiency

- ❧ There have been epidemic increases in multiple CHCs, especially obesity and type 2 diabetes.
- ❧ Annual estimated costs from inactivity in the U.S. include:

Key Points: Physical Activity Deficiency (*Continued*)

At least $150 billion per year in direct and indirect healthcare costs
At least 334,000 premature deaths per year
Nonquantifiable human suffering inflicted by multiple CHCs.

Suggested Reading

1. Hoffman C, Rice D, Sung HY. Persons with chronic conditions. Their prevalence and costs. JAMA 276: 1473–1479, 1996.
2. Hahn RA, Teutsch SM, Rothenberg RB, Marks JS. Excess deaths from nine chronic diseases in the United States in 1986. JAMA 264: 2654–2659, 1990.
3. Boyle JP, Honeycutt AA, Narayan KM, et al. Projection of diabetes burden through 2050: Impact of changing demography and disease prevalence in the U.S. Diabetes Care 24(11): 1936–1940, 2001.
4. Flegal KM, Troiano RP. Changes in the distribution of body mass index of adults and children in the US population. Int J Obes Relat Metab Disord 24(7): 807–818, 2000.
5. Mokdad AH, Bowman BA, Ford ES, et al. The continuing epidemics of obesity and diabetes in the United States. JAMA 286:1195–1200, 2001.
6. Allison DB, Fontaine KR, Manson JE, et al. Annual deaths attributable to obesity in the United States. JAMA 282(16): 1530–1538, 1999.
7. Must A, Spadano J, Coakley EH, et al. The disease burden associated with over-weight and obesity. JAMA 282:1523–1529, 1999.
8. Jung RT. Obesity as a disease. Br Med Bull 53(2): 307–321, 1997.
9. Campion EW. The oldest old. New Engl J Med 330: 1819–1820, 1994.
10. Pratt M, Macera CA, Wang G. Higher direct medical costs associated with physical inactvitiy. Phys Sportsmed 28: 63–70, 2000.
11. Wang G, et al. Inactivity-associated medical costs among US adults with arthritis. Arthritis Rheum Arthritis Care Res 45: 439–445, 2001.
12. McGinnis JM, Foege WH. Actual causes of death in the United States. JAMA 270: 2017–2022, 1993.
13. Zimmet P, Alberti KG, Shaw J. Global and societal implications of the diabetes epidemic. Nature 414: 782–787, 2001.

Childrens' Health Endangered

chapter

5

Pediatric Obesity

Inactivity severely endangers the health of our children. Pediatric obesity, for example, is associated with a frightening number of significant health disorders. Overweight children/adolescents are not as healthy as lean children/adolescents, and there is a greater prevalence of various disorders in the former (Tables 5–1 and 5–2).

TABLE 5–1. Comprehensive List of Morbidities With Increased Prevalence* in Obese Children/Adolescents	
Organ System/Performance	**Disorder**
Cardiovascular	Hypertension
Endocrine	Decreased growth hormone, increased IGF-I Dyslipidemia Insulin resistance PCOS Pubertal advancement
Gastrointestinal	Gallstones Steatohepatitis
Neurological	Pseudotumor
Orthopedic	Blount's disease Slipped capital femoral epiphysis
Pulmonary	Asthma Sleep abnormality/central hypoventilation
Socioeconomic	Downward economic mobility Low self-esteem in adolescence Poor school performance
*In the short term IGF = insulin-like growth factor Data from references 1–8	

TABLE 5–2.	Comprehensive List of Morbidities With Increased Prevalence in Adulthood Due To Childhood/Adolescent Obesity
Morbidity/Mortality	**Disorder**
Morbidity	Arthritis
	Atherosclerosis cerebrovascular disorder
	Colorectal cancer
	Coronary heart disease
	Gout
	Loss of activities of daily living
	Type 2 diabetes
Mortality	All-cause
	Cardiovascular
Data from reference 1.	

Certain disorders, such as Blount's disease, are closely associated with obesity in children (Fig. 5–1). Morbidly obese children (BMI > 97th percentile for age) have increased preponderance of steatohepatitis and obesity hypoventilation syndrome, compared to lean children (BMI < 75th percentile) of the same age (Fig. 5–2). The percentage of total hospital discharges of obesity-related disorders in youths aged 6–17 years old doubled, in a recent 20-year period (Fig. 5–3).[4]

Figure 5–1. Percentage of obese children having various comorbid disorders. (Adapted from Must, A Strauss RS. Risks and consequences of childhood and adolescent obesity. Int J Obes Relat Metab Disord 23 Suppl 2:S2–11, 1999.)

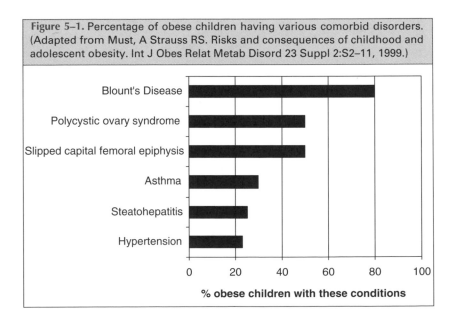

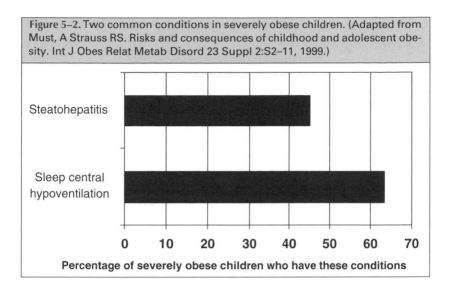

Figure 5–2. Two common conditions in severely obese children. (Adapted from Must, A Strauss RS. Risks and consequences of childhood and adolescent obesity. Int J Obes Relat Metab Disord 23 Suppl 2:S2–11, 1999.)

Increased Risk of Chronic Health Conditions in Adulthood

Most overweight children/adolescents already have **cardiovascular disease** (CVD) risk factors. Approximately 60% of overweight 5- to 10-year-old children and overweight 11- to 17-year-old adolescents already have one associated biochemical or clinical cardiovascular risk

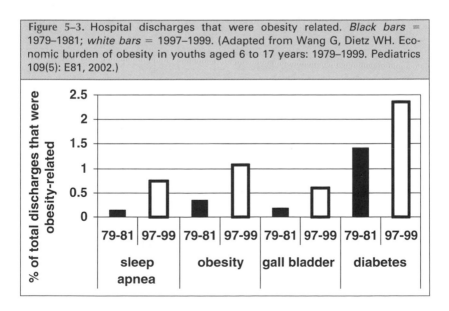

Figure 5–3. Hospital discharges that were obesity related. *Black bars =* 1979–1981; *white bars* = 1997–1999. (Adapted from Wang G, Dietz WH. Economic burden of obesity in youths aged 6 to 17 years: 1979–1999. Pediatrics 109(5): E81, 2002.)

factor (such as hyperlipidemia, hypertension, or increased insulin levels), and 25% have two or more.[5] Overweight schoolchildren (defined by Freedman et al as having a BMI > 95th percentile) had anywhere from two to twelve times the chance of having CVD risk factors as compared to schoolchildren with < 85th percentile BMI (Fig. 5–4). For example, an overweight child is two times as likely to have total serum cholesterol of 200 mg/dL than is a lean child.

Coronary artery disease was found among post-adolescent U.S. soldiers (18–21 years old) killed in action in Korea (JAMA 152:1090–1093, 1953). The American Heart Association (AHA) recently stated that the pathological data *proves* that atherosclerosis begins in childhood, and that the extent of atherosclerotic plaque development in children and young adults correlates with the same risk factors identified in adults (see Fig 5–4). The AHA asserted that it is eminently reasonable to initiate healthful lifestyle training in childhood to promote improved cardiovascular health in adult life.

Risk factors for the **metabolic syndrome** (see Chapter 12) are defined in the study by Freedman et al[5] as triglycerides > 130 mg/dL, low-density lipoproteins > 130 mg/dL, high-density lipoproteins < 35 mg/dL, insulin > 95th percentile, and either systolic or diastolic blood pressure > 95th percentile. Twenty-two percent of all children with one risk factor

Figure 5–4. Odds ratio that an obese child has of exceeding the threshold for CVD risk factors. (Adapted from Freedman DS, Dietz WH, Srinivasan SR, Berenson GS: The relation of overweight to cardiovascular risk factors among children and adolescents: The Bogalusa Heart Study. Pediatrics 103(6):1175–1182, 1999.)

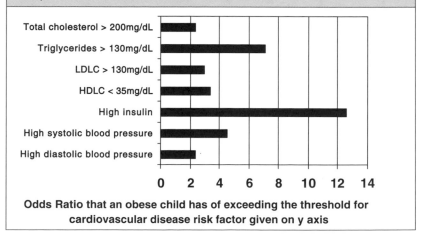

Odds Ratio that an obese child has of exceeding the threshold for cardiovascular disease risk factor given on y axis

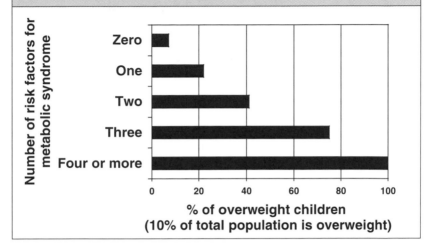

Figure 5-5. The link between metabolic syndrome and obesity. (Adapted from Freedman DS, Dietz WH, Srinivasan SR, Berenson GS: The relation of overweight to cardiovascular risk factors among children and adolescents: The Bogalusa Heart Study. Pediatrics 103(6):1175–1182, 1999.)

for the metabolic syndrome are overweight; 100% of all children with all four risk factors for the metabolic syndrome are overweight (Fig. 5–5).

Obese children/adolescents already have risk factors for **type 2 diabetes,** and some have clinically overt type 2 diabetes.[6] Children (4- to 10-year-olds) with BMI > 30 kg/m² have increased fasting blood insulin (Fig. 5–6). Hyperinsulinemia is the harbinger of insulin resistance, which is believed to be one of the major initiators of the metabolic syndrome cascade.

Some adolescents with BMI ≥ 35 kg/m² already have insulin resistance and elevated fasting C-peptide levels (Fig. 5–7), both of which are manifestations of overt type 2 diabetes.

Given these alarming trends, it is reasonable to expect many adolescents with type 2 diabetes to present with microvascular and macrovascular complications of diabetes as early as young adulthood. This has indeed been the case, as shown by Young et al.[7]

Overweight/obese children and adolescents with the highest BMIs are more likely to have **clustering of factors** in metabolic syndrome when they are adults (Fig. 5–8). In one study,[8] 15% of children with the highest BMIs had clustering of metabolic syndrome factors (i.e., high fasting insulin, systolic or mean blood pressures, and total cholesterol/triglycerides to HDL-cholesterol ratio) 11 years later.

Moreover, being overweight/obese as children/adolescents was associated with a disproportionately high prevalence of adverse health effects

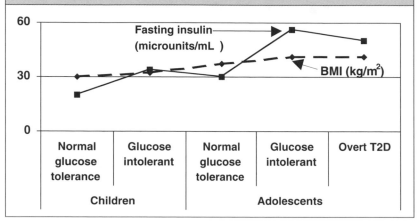

Figure 5–6. Diabetes and obesity (*dashed line* = BMI; *solid line* = fasting insulin levels). *T2D* = type 2 diabetes. (Adapted from Sinha R, Fisch G, Teague B, et al. Prevalence of impaired glucose tolerance among children and adolescents with marked obesity. New Engl J Med 346:802–810, 2002.)

that were *independent of adult body weight* 55 years later in men and women (Fig 5–9).[9] The follow-up to the Harvard Growth Study by Must et al[9] also found that overweight male and female adolescents had greater difficulty with activities of daily living (ADL) later in life (Fig. 5–10). Also, being an overweight adolescent male significantly pre-

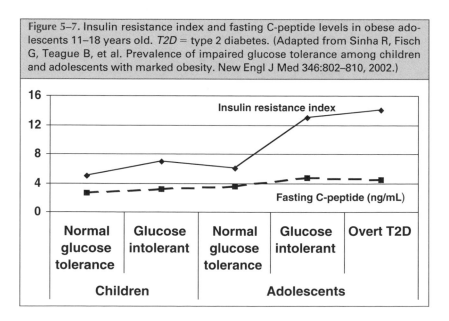

Figure 5–7. Insulin resistance index and fasting C-peptide levels in obese adolescents 11–18 years old. *T2D* = type 2 diabetes. (Adapted from Sinha R, Fisch G, Teague B, et al. Prevalence of impaired glucose tolerance among children and adolescents with marked obesity. New Engl J Med 346:802–810, 2002.)

Figure 5-8. Association between high BMI in childhood and clustering of metabolic syndrome factors in adulthood. (Adapted from Srinivasan SR, Myers L, Berenson GS: Predictability of childhood adiposity and insulin for developing insulin resistance syndrome (syndrome X) in young adulthood: The Bogalusa Heart Study. Diabetes 51(1):204–209, 2002.)

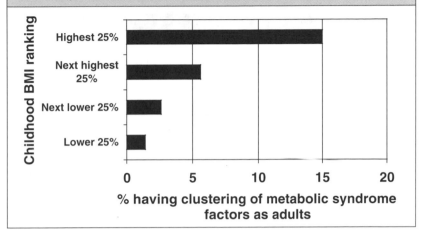

dicted an increased relative risk of death, 55 years later (Fig. 5–11). *Overweight adolescent females had no such increased mortality risk!*

An obese child has a high probability of becoming an obese adult.[10] An odds ratio of 2 or 20 (Fig. 5–12) means that the obese child has twice or 24 times the chance of being an obese adult, compared to a non-

Figure 5-9. Relative risk of adverse health conditions 55 years after being an overweight child. (Adapted from Must A, et al: Long-term morbidity and mortality of overweight adolescents. A follow-up of the Harvard Growth Study of 1922 to 1935. N Engl J Med 327:1350–1355, 1992.)

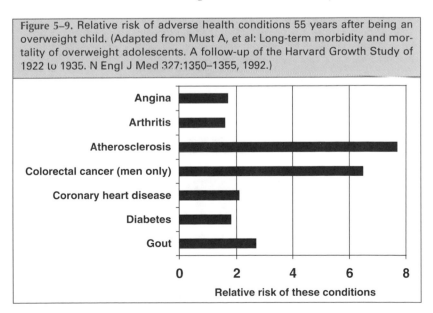

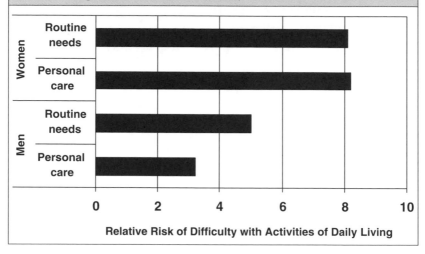

Figure 5–10. Relative risk of difficulty with daily living 55 yrs after being an overweight child. (Adapted from Must A, et al: Long-term morbidity and mortality of overweight adolescents. A follow-up of the Harvard Growth Study of 1922 to 1935. N Engl J Med 327:1350–1355, 1992.)

obese child. In fact, the incidence of childhood obesity doubled in a 13-year period (Fig. 5–13). What changed from 1976–1980 to 1988–1994 to cause this dramatic doubling of obesity in U.S. children?

The answer is found in **lifestyle.** Our children are much more physi-

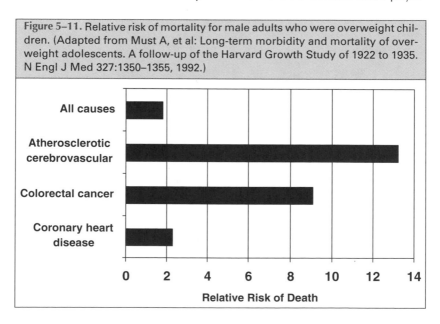

Figure 5–11. Relative risk of mortality for male adults who were overweight children. (Adapted from Must A, et al: Long-term morbidity and mortality of overweight adolescents. A follow-up of the Harvard Growth Study of 1922 to 1935. N Engl J Med 327:1350–1355, 1992.)

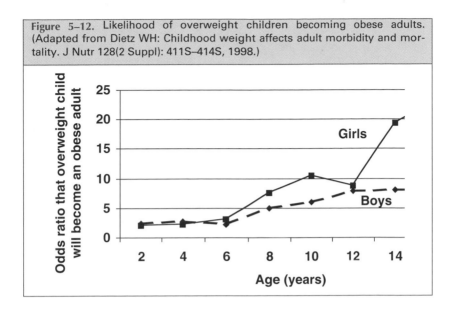

Figure 5–12. Likelihood of overweight children becoming obese adults. (Adapted from Dietz WH: Childhood weight affects adult morbidity and mortality. J Nutr 128(2 Suppl): 411S–414S, 1998.)

cally inactive than previous generations. The increase in obesity is due to environmental changes—such as a marked decline in physical activity *and* a concomitant increase in sedentary behavior and ingestion of high-calorie foods and drinks—affecting existing susceptibility genes.

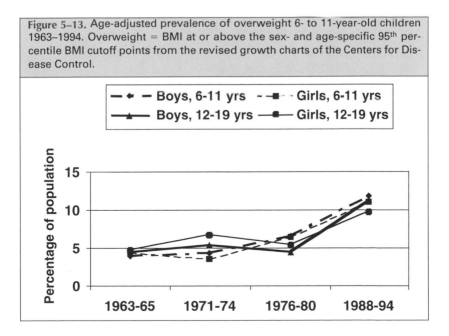

Figure 5–13. Age-adjusted prevalence of overweight 6- to 11-year-old children 1963–1994. Overweight = BMI at or above the sex- and age-specific 95th percentile BMI cutoff points from the revised growth charts of the Centers for Disease Control.

Summary of the Effects of Childhood Obesity

The disease consequences of pediatric obesity are vast. The overweight/obese child/adolescent is at increased risk of disorders that require immediate pediatric assessment and intervention (see Chapter 10, Physical Activity Prescription and Weight Loss Counseling). Also, overweight/obesity prematurely initiates multiple chronic health conditions in children/adolescents who are then more likely to manifest overt clinical symptoms as early as late adolescence and young adulthood. The assertion can be made that the disease consequences of childhood obesity are likely to result in an increased prevalence of disorders in the general population 55 years later.

Most childhood obesity is *not* the result of new mutations in existing genes. Rather, changes in the lifestyle of our children are initiating the expression of metabolic disorders such as obesity.

Children are too young to decide whether to be physically inactive or not, and to fully appreciate or comprehend the devastating consequences of the multiple premature chronic health problems that could await them as adults, if they continue to remain physically inactive. For precisely this reason, it is a prime obligation of the healthcare profession to "immunize" children (much the same way we already routinely do for childhood infections) against physical inactivity and sedentary lifestyles, and the associated disease consequences.

Primary Prevention of Pediatric Obesity

Decrease Sedentary Activity

Sedentary time for children has increased in the past few decades. This shift from active to passive play has resulted in fewer calories expended, and more of these unused calories stored as fat. Studies have shown that children spent more time in physical activities and less time watching TV in the 1950s than they did in the 1990s.

- In the 1950s, children spent only 86 minutes per day in front of the TV or engaged in sedentary activities (Fig. 5–14).
- In the 1990s, children's TV watching time (used as a surrogate for sedentary time) *tripled,* averaging 4–4.5 hours of TV watching per day!

Although no quantitative data that is comparable to TV watching across decades was found to document the generally accepted idea that there has been a progressive decline in children's physical activity, comparing children's daily routines in the 1950s to those in the 21st century amply supports this notion (Table 5–3).

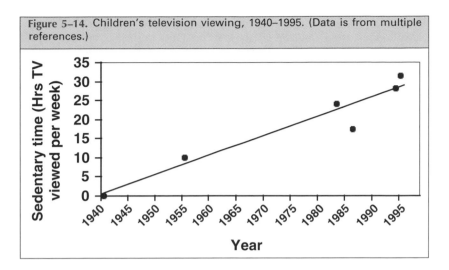

Figure 5–14. Children's television viewing, 1940–1995. (Data is from multiple references.)

The American Academy of Pediatrics (AAP) has produced guidelines for children's TV viewing:

- Children younger than 2 years old should watch no television.
- Children 2 years and older should watch < 2 hours of television per day.

However, the reality is that these AAP-recommended viewing hours are exceeded by 17% for ages 0–11 months and 48% for ages 12–23 months[12] (Fig. 5–15). Unfortunately, children's TV viewing increases from age 3 to age 8, at which point the AAP guidelines are exceeded by twice the limit (Fig. 5–16).

Longitudinal analysis[12] shows that the amount of TV viewing in early childhood is directly proportional to that viewed at school age. Thus,

TABLE 5–3. Comparison of Children's Activities, 1950s and 21st Century	
1950s	**21st Century**
Walking or cycling to school	Bus or car to school
Physical education	Reduced or no physical education
Recess	Reduced or no recess
Physical chores outside of school	Automated chores
Physical play time	Viewing TV, computer games, internet
Access to playgrounds without parental supervision	Adult supervision required for activities outside the home
Spontaneous play	More structured play requiring transportation to play area

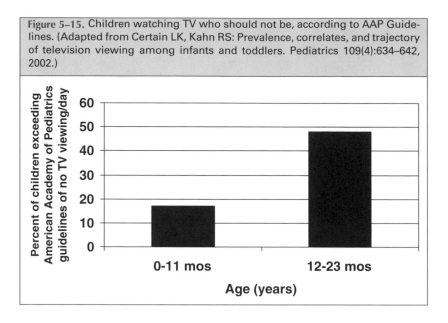

Figure 5–15. Children watching TV who should not be, according to AAP Guidelines. (Adapted from Certain LK, Kahn RS: Prevalence, correlates, and trajectory of television viewing among infants and toddlers. Pediatrics 109(4):634–642, 2002.)

preventive measures against excessive TV watching must begin *before* the age of 2, as other studies[13] suggest a causal relationship between school-age TV viewing and obesity and aggression. Remarkably, in 10- to 15-year-old children/adolescents, the odds of being overweight quadruple and the odds of regaining lost weight are eight times greater

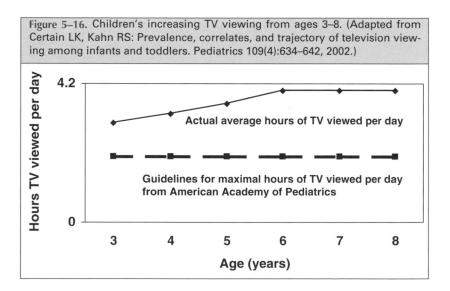

Figure 5–16. Children's increasing TV viewing from ages 3–8. (Adapted from Certain LK, Kahn RS: Prevalence, correlates, and trajectory of television viewing among infants and toddlers. Pediatrics 109(4):634–642, 2002.)

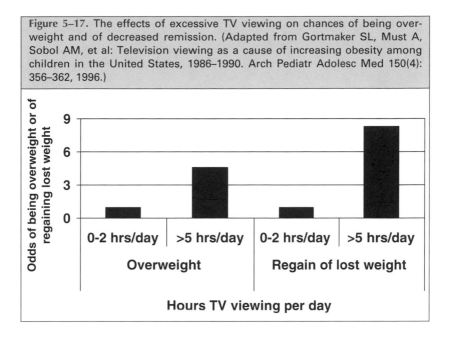

Figure 5–17. The effects of excessive TV viewing on chances of being overweight and of decreased remission. (Adapted from Gortmaker SL, Must A, Sobol AM, et al: Television viewing as a cause of increasing obesity among children in the United States, 1986–1990. Arch Pediatr Adolesc Med 150(4): 356–362, 1996.)

with excessive TV viewing[13] (Fig. 5–17). Thus, reductions in TV viewing time could significantly decrease childhood obesity.

Improve Nutrition

Consider the concept of **caloric balance** (see Chapter 7, Caloric Balance and Expenditure, for more detailed information). Body mass is the balance between calories in and calories out. In a non-growing individual, caloric imbalance is the only way to alter body mass, and the only way to change caloric balance is to eat more and/or move less.

In *growing* children, the caloric balance has to do more than maintain body weight; it has to allow normal increases in height and organ sizes with age, but not be excessive so that overweight or obesity develops. If BMI exceeds the 85th percentile, it is likely that caloric balance is lacking for the child/adolescent.

Primary prevention of childhood overweight and progression to obesity demands that strict attention be paid to growth charts and relative percentile of body weights. Factors in the family, school, and community environments that affect food intake and physical activity levels must all be examined. Parent's body habitus could be considered a genetic barometer of a child's genetic predisposition to become obese, and aggressive early interventions could be instituted.

Interestingly, during childrens' TV programs in the UK, 62.5% of advertising time was devoted to foodstuffs (primetime [evening hours] only devoted 18.4% of advertising time to foods). Of the time spent advertising foods during childrens' TV programs, 73.4% was devoted to products high in sugar (18.6% of primetime advertising featured high-sugar products). These observations replicate those in the U.S., where half of 21.3 commercials per hour viewed in childrens' TV programming were food advertisements (91% of which advertised foods high in fat, sugar, and/or salt).[14] Watching TV is often associated with increased snacking (increased caloric intake), and children are being encouraged to eat fattening foods.

Primary and Secondary Prevention More Effective Than Tertiary Prevention

As childhood obesity was preventable 50 years ago as evidenced by its low incidence, our commonsense conclusion is that it can also be prevented now—by instituting lifestyle modifications. Primary prevention of childhood obesity is not a choice; it is *mandatory* on the grounds that:

- Children are too immature to make life-altering decisions on their own.
- Physicians must protect children's health and ensure that no harm is done to them.

Although behavioral modifications can attenuate existing childhood obesity, they are costly in terms of time, money, and child safety. Moreover, a significant number of parents cannot afford basic medical care, much less costly tertiary interventions. Thus, we plead for primary prevention. Limitations on TV viewing and/or elimination of high-sugar drinks are behavioral modifications for children < 5 years of age that are under the direct control of parents. The alternative is paying providers for tertiary prevention to lose weight, which on the whole has a low success rate.

Parents, daycare providers, and grandparents must take charge and limit TV viewing time to counter powerful commercial marketing interests, and must stop giving children high-sugar drinks. Most young children mind their parents, and they can be told to go play. Children need access to a room/playground/play area near their home for active play, which will allow them to expend calories. All healthcare professionals should inform parents of the AAP Guidelines regarding TV viewing time.

We understand that the social and environmental factors that have produced the epidemic of childhood obesity are complex and not easily altered. This is why we suggest that, at a minimum, healthcare professionals promote the AAP Guidelines. This would not abolish 100%

of childhood obesity, but it would put a big dent in this gargantuan problem.

Suggested Reading

1. Must A, Strauss RS. Risks and consequences of childhood and adolescent obesity. Int J Obes Relat Metab Disord 23 Suppl 2:S2–11, 1999.
2. Caprio S, Tamborlane WV. Metabolic impact of obesity in childhood. Endocrinol Metab Clin North Am 28:731–747, 1999.
3. Yanovski JA. Pediatric obesity. Rev Endocr Metab Disord 2:371–383, 2001.
4. Wang G, Dietz WH. Economic burden of obesity in youths aged 6 to 17 years: 1979–1999. Pediatrics 109(5): E81–1, 2002.
5. Freedman DS, Dietz WH, Srinivasan SR, Berenson GS. The relation of overweight to cardiovascular risk factors among children and adolescents: The Bogalusa Heart Study. Pediatrics 103 (6): 1175–1182, 1999.
6. Sinha R, Fisch G, Teague B, et al. Prevalence of impaired glucose tolerance among children and adolescents with marked obesity. New Engl J Med 346:802–810, 2002.
7. Young TK, Dean HJ, Flett B, Wood-Steiman P. Childhood obesity in a population at high risk for type 2 diabetes. J Pediatr. 136(3): 365–369, 2000.
8. Srinivasan SR, Myers L, Berenson GS. Predictability of childhood adiposity and in-sulin for developing insulin resistance syndrome (syndrome X) in young adulthood: The Bogalusa Heart Study Diabetes 51(1):204–209, 2002.
9. Must A, et al: Long-term morbidity and mortality of overweight adolescents. A follow-up of the Harvard Growth Study of 1922 to 1935. N Engl J Med 327:1350–1355, 1992.
10. Dietz WH. Childhood weight affects adult morbidity and mortality. J Nutr 128(2 Suppl): 411S–414S, 1998.
11. Mokdad AH, Bowman BA, Ford ES, et al. The continuing epidemics of obesity and diabetes in the United States. JAMA 286: 1195–1200, 2001.
12. Certain LK, Kahn RS. Prevalence, correlates, and trajectory of television viewing among infants and toddlers. Pediatrics 109(4):634–642, 2002.
13. Gortmaker SL, Must A, Sobol AM, et al. Television viewing as a cause of increasing obesity among children in the United States, 1986–1990. Arch Pediatr Adolesc Med 150(4): 356–362, 1996.
14. Taras HL, Gage M. Advertised foods on children's television. Arch Pediatr Adolesc Med 149: 649–652, 1995.

SECTION II
The Means To Action

chapter
6

Health Benefits of Physical Activity

The Power of Environmental Factors

Environmental factors, including physical inactivity, are responsible for most of the increase in chronic health conditions (Fig. 6–1).

Scandinavian Twin Studies. Data from 44,788 pairs of twins listed in the Swedish, Danish, and Finnish twin registries showed that inherited

Figure 6–1. The contribution of environmental factors to disease. (Adapted from Lichtenstein P, Holm NV, Verkasalo PK, et al. Environmental and heritable factors in the causation of cancer—Analyses of cohorts of twins from Sweden, Denmark, and Finland. N Engl J Med 343:78–85, 2000.)

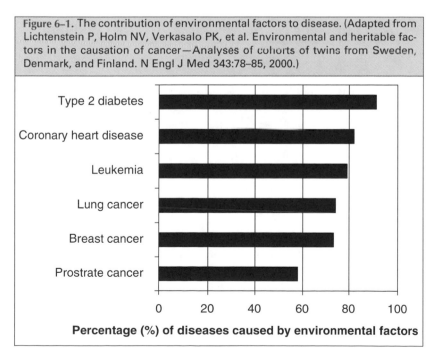

Percentage (%) of diseases caused by environmental factors

genetic factors make only a minor contribution to susceptibility to most types of neoplasms.[1] This study concluded that the environment has the principal role in causing most types of sporadic cancer.

Harvard Nurses Health Studies. A low-risk pattern of behavior was defined as:

- BMI < 25 kg/m^2
- A diet high in cereal fiber and polyunsaturated fat and low in trans fat and glycemic load (diet affects blood glucose level)
- Engagement in moderate-to-vigorous physical activity for at least half an hour per day
- No current smoking
- Consumption of at least half an alcoholic beverage per day (in the population studied, only 1.2% of the women reported drinking > 45 g alcohol per day, so an upper limit could not be established).

These low-risk behaviors offered primary prevention for type 2 diabetes and coronary artery disease. Ninety-one percent of diabetes cases[2] and 82% of coronary events[3] in the study cohort could be attributed to habits and forms of behavior that did not conform to the low-risk pattern. Therefore, among women in the Harvard Nurses Health Study, adherence to lifestyle guidelines for diet, physical activity, and smoking was associated with a very low risk of diabetes and coronary heart disease.

Reduced Prevalence of Many Chronic Health Conditions

Moderate physical activity ($\geq$ 30 min of brisk walking per day) reduces the incidence of many chronic health conditions (CHCs; Fig. 6–2), as compared to a sedentary lifestyle (< 30 min walking per day).[4–6] Multiple consensus statements from several groups support this data. Examples include:

- The Centers for Disease Control and Prevention (CDC) and American College of Sport Medicine (ACSM) recommendation on physical activity and public health,[7] which stated that if sedentary individuals adopted only moderate increases in physical activity, public health would benefit by a reduction in chronic diseases. Activities such as running marathons are not needed to gain this benefit.
- The Surgeon General's Report on *Physical Activity and Health* published in 1996, which asserted that "Physical activity of the type that improves cardiovascular endurance reduces the risk of developing or dying from cardiovascular disease, hypertension, colon cancer, and type 2 diabetes and improves mental health. Findings are suggestive that endurance-type physical activity may reduce the risk of developing obesity, osteoporosis, and depression and may improve psychological well-being and quality of life. There is promising ev-

Figure 6–2. Moderate physical activity benefits many chronic health conditions.

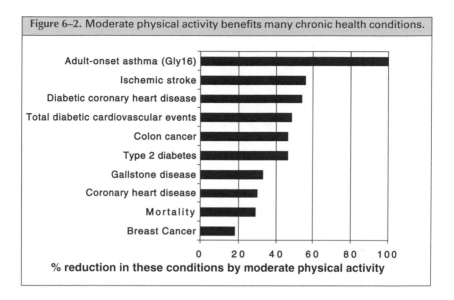

% reduction in these conditions by moderate physical activity

idence that muscle strengthening (resistance) exercise reduces the risk of falling and fractures among the elderly."

- A Statement for Health Professionals by the Committee on Exercise and Cardiac Rehabilitation of the Council on Clinical Cardiology, American Heart Association, which declared that physical inactivity is a risk factor for coronary artery disease and that physicians have the opportunity and responsibility to promote regular physical activity either personally or via delegation to other members of the healthcare team. If delegation is selected, the physician should initially set and support the physical activity agenda.[9]

- A consensus statement from an ACSM-sponsored symposium, which stated that regular physical activity is associated with a reduction in all-cause mortality, fatal and nonfatal total cardiovascular disease, coronary heart disease, obesity, type 2 diabetes mellitus, colon cancer, osteoporosis, physical frailty, and depressive illness.[10]

- An article by Jeffrey Koplan, Director of the CDC in 2001, which says, in part: " . . . restoring physical activity to our daily routines is crucial to the future reduction of diabetes and obesity in the U.S. population."[11]

- An Executive Order issued by President George W. Bush on June 20, 2002—

  Section 1. Policy. This order is issued consistent with the following findings and principles:

  (a) Growing scientific evidence indicates that an increasing number of Americans are suffering from negligible physical activity, poor dietary habits, insufficient utilization of preventive health screenings, and engaging in risky behaviors such as abuse of alcohol, tobacco, and drugs.

(b) Existing information on the importance of appropriate physical activity, diet, preventive health screenings, and avoiding harmful substances is often not received by the public, or, if received, is not acted on sufficiently.

(c) Individuals of all ages, locations, and levels of personal fitness can benefit from some level of appropriate physical activity, dietary guidance, preventive health screening, and making healthy choices.

(d) While personal fitness is an individual responsibility, the Federal Government may, within the authority and funds otherwise available, expand the opportunities for individuals to empower themselves to improve their general health. Such opportunities may include improving the flow of information about personal fitness, assisting in the utilization of that information, increasing the accessibility of resources for physical activity, and reducing barriers to achieving good personal fitness.

- A 2002 recommendation by The Institute of Medicine of the National Academy of Sciences stated that 60 minutes of moderate, daily physical activity are required to maintain body mass index at 18.5–25 kg/m^2 and to receive additional, weight-independent health benefits.

Summary of the Clinical Evidence

Several landmark clinical studies and trials have showed that moderate-intensity physical activity reduces the prevalence of many chronic health conditions (Table 6–1).

Harvard Nurses Health Study.[12–14] The Harvard Nurses' Health Study was initiated in 1976, with 121,700 female registered nurses 30 to 55 years old. After women who reported a diagnosis of CVD or cancer at baseline were excluded, the population for analysis comprised 72,488 women 40 to 65 years old in 1986. Participants were asked the average amount of time they spent per week doing moderate or vigorous recreational activities. They were also asked about their usual walking pace, specified as easy (< 2 mph), moderate (2.0–2.9 mph), brisk (3.0–3.9 mph), or very brisk (≥ 4 mph). Walking requires an energy expenditure of only 2.0–4.5 METs (≥ 2- to 4.5-fold increase from resting metabolic rate), depending on pace; therefore, it was considered to be a moderate-intensity activity. Any physical activity requiring > 6 METs was consid-

TABLE 6–1. Physical Activity Benefits Health in Almost Every Disease Category

Disorder Affected	Effect of Increased Activity	Evidence Category*
All-cause mortality	Decrease	C
All-cause CVD and CHD	Decrease	C
Blood pressure	Decrease	A
Colon cancer	Decrease	C
Depression	Decrease	B
Diabetes (type 2)	Decrease	A
HDL-cholesterol	Increase	B
Insulin resistance	Decrease (lasts for only 3–4 days after a single exercise bout)	A
Osteoporosis	Decrease	B
Triglycerides (blood)	Decrease	C
Body weight	Decrease	A

CVD = cardiovascular disease, CHD = coronary heart disease
*Definitions of evidence categories:
Category A—evidence from endpoints of well-designed randomized clinical trial (RCTs) that provide a consistent pattern of findings. Category A thus requires substantial numbers of studies involving a substantial number of participants.
Category B—evidence is from endpoints of intervention that include only a limited number of RCTs, post hoc or subgroup analysis of RCTs, or meta-analysis of RCTs. Category B pertains when few randomized trials exist, they are small, and the trial results are somewhat inconsistent.
Category C—evidence is from outcomes of uncontrolled or nonrandomized trials or from observational studies.

ered to be vigorous. **Major outcome/conclusions:** The data from these studies conclusively demonstrated that physical activity of moderate intensity and duration (i.e., brisk walking for at least 30 minutes) is associated with *substantial* reductions in the—

- Incidence of coronary events
- Risk of total and ischemic stroke (in a dose-response manner)
- Risk of type 2 diabetes.

Subpopulation of Harvard Nurses Health Study.[2,12] This study included 5125 women who, on any questionnaire from 1976 to 1992, reported having physician-diagnosed diabetes mellitus and being 30 years of age or older at disease onset (a working definition for inclusion in the study). Women who reported a history of CHD (including myocardial infarction, angina, or coronary revascularization), stroke, or cancer on or before the 1980 questionnaire (when physical activity was first assessed) were excluded at baseline. **Major outcome/conclusions:** Among women with diabetes, increased physical activity, including regular walking, was associated with *substantially* reduced risk for cardiovascular events.

Diabetes Prevention Study, Finland.[16] In this study 522 middle-aged, overweight subjects (172 men and 350 women; mean age 55 yrs; mean BMI 31 kg/m²), with impaired glucose tolerance were randomly assigned to either the lifestyle intervention group or the control group. **Major outcome/conclusions:** The risk of diabetes was reduced by 58% (P < 0.001) in the lifestyle intervention group. The reduction in the incidence of diabetes was directly associated with changes in lifestyle. Thus, type 2 diabetes can be prevented by changes in the lifestyle of high-risk subjects.

Diabetes Prevention Program, U.S.[15] This clinical trial involved 3234 nondiabetic persons with elevated fasting and post-load plasma glucose concentrations. They were randomly assigned to placebo, metformin (850 mg twice daily), or a lifestyle-modification program. **Major outcome/conclusions:** Lifestyle intervention was *twice as effective* as drug treatment in preventing overt clinical type 2 diabetes in patients with glucose intolerance (i.e., "prediabetic"patients; Fig. 6–3).

The U.S. Diabetes Prevention Program Trial was unique because of its large sample size and great inclusion of ethnic minorities (50% of participants). Of note, none of the participants had overt clinical type 2 diabetes at the start of the study; they were "pre-diabetic." The goals for the participants assigned to the intensive lifestyle intervention were to achieve and maintain a weight reduction of at least 7% of initial body weight through a healthy, low-calorie, low-fat diet and to engage in physical activity of moderate intensity, such as brisk walking, for at least 150 minutes per week. A 16-lesson curriculum taught by case managers on a one-to-one basis covering diet, exercise, and behavior modification

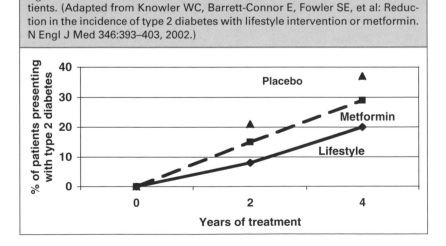

Figure 6–3. Results of three interventions in glucose intolerant (prediabetic) patients. (Adapted from Knowler WC, Barrett-Connor E, Fowler SE, et al: Reduction in the incidence of type 2 diabetes with lifestyle intervention or metformin. N Engl J Med 346:393–403, 2002.)

was designed to help the participants achieve these goals. Subsequent individual sessions (usually monthly) and group sessions with the case managers were designed to reinforce the behavioral changes.

- Both lifestyle modification and metformin treatment prevented the progression of glucose intolerance to overt clinical diabetes, compared to placebo.
- However, lifestyle modification was *twice as effective* as metformin (58% vs. 31%) in reducing the occurrence of type 2 diabetes in "prediabetic" (glucose intolerant) patients.
- Additionally, participants assigned to lifestyle intervention lost 5.6 kg body weight, while the metformin and placebo groups lost 0.1 and 2.1 kg, respectively.
- Though the reduction in the average fasting plasma glucose concentration was similar in the lifestyle intervention and metformin groups, lifestyle intervention had a greater decrease in glycosylated hemoglobin and resulted in more participants having normal postprandial glucose values at follow-up, compared to the group treated with metformin.
- To prevent one case of diabetes during a period of 3 years, only 6.9 persons would have to participate in the lifestyle-intervention program, compared to 13.9 persons with metformin.

Benefits of Cardiovascular Fitness

Low levels of cardiovascular fitness are associated with an increased risk of dying. Myers et al[17] found that, of the men who had had a normal exercise-stress test and no history of CVD 14 years earlier, 57% died in the group who started out with lowest maximal aerobic capacity (< 5 METs), compared to only 17% deaths in those with twice the maximal aerobic capacity (> 8 MET; Fig. 6–4).

Maximal aerobic capacity is not fixed; physical inactivity lowers it. Conversely, physical activity slows decline of maximal aerobic capacity due to aging and, if vigorous enough, can actually raise the level of maximal aerobic capacity. Subjects with < 5 METs aerobic capacity have 4.5 times greater risk of dying than those with > 8 METs aerobic capacity. This is not a trivial difference! Myers et al[17] found that every 1 MET increase in treadmill performance was associated with a 12% improvement in survival, which emphasizes that aerobic exercise capacity can be used as a relatively strong prognostic value for survival.

The terms "maximal aerobic capacity" and "cardiovascular fitness" are roughly interchangeable because the capacity to use oxygen to fuel work is limited by the ability of: (1) the heart to pump blood, (2) the cardiovascular system to deliver the arterialized blood to working skeletal

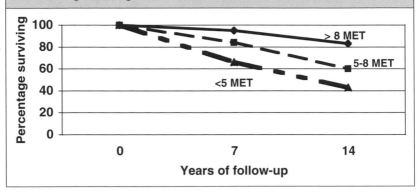

Figure 6–4. Association of low levels of cardiovascular fitness with increased risk of dying. MET = metabolic equivalent of the task. The greater the MET value, the greater the aerobic capacity. (Adapted from Myers J, Prakash M, Froelicher V, et al. Exercise capacity and mortality among men referred for exercise testing. New Engl J Med 346:793–801, 2002.)

muscle, and (3) the muscle's enzymatic machinery to use the delivered oxygen to convert glucose and fatty acids into high energy phosphates (ATP) to support muscle contraction.

Interestingly, in a study by Blair et al,[18] survival was found to significantly improve when unfit men became fit (Fig. 6–5). Some of the subjects began physical training in the eighth year of the study. These results show that becoming physically fit is a potent and highly effective mode of primary prevention.

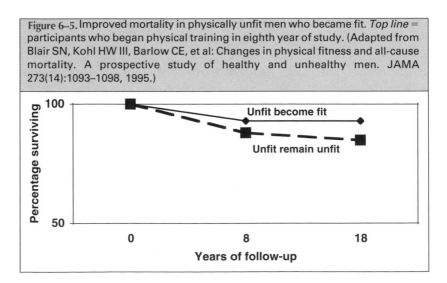

Figure 6–5. Improved mortality in physically unfit men who became fit. *Top line =* participants who began physical training in eighth year of study. (Adapted from Blair SN, Kohl HW III, Barlow CE, et al: Changes in physical fitness and all-cause mortality. A prospective study of healthy and unhealthy men. JAMA 273(14):1093–1098, 1995.)

Benefits of Cardiovascular Fitness Extend Across All Body Weight Classifications

Low cardiovascular fitness increases the risk of dying in normal weight, overweight, and obese men (Fig. 6–6).[19] Low cardiovascular fitness is more hazardous to health than smoking. As ~70% of adults in the U.S. are sedentary and only ~25% of adults in the U.S. smoke, *the absolute number of deaths from being physically unfit should vastly exceed that of smoking once the proper studies are done.* Currently, our estimates do not support this extrapolation; they show slightly fewer deaths from being sedentary than from smoking. Our estimate of annual deaths in the U.S. from physical inactivity is 334,000, while the CDC indicates that there are 430,000 deaths from tobacco each year.

Cardiovascular Fitness Effects on Chronic Health Conditions

The relationship between cardiovascular (aerobic) fitness and mortality extends to many chronic health conditions.

Cardiovascular disease:
- Low aerobic fitness increases the risk of dying in patients with CVD[17] (Fig. 6–7).
- The relative risk of dying in patients with CVD is 4.5 times greater in the lowest aerobically fit group (1.0–4.9 METs), compared to the highest aerobically fit group (> 10.7 METs).

Figure 6–6. Low cardiovascular fitness ("unfit," *white bars*) increases the relative risk of all-cause mortality in all weight categories compared to fit (*black bars*). Furthermore, the increased risk of dying due to low physical fitness is greater than the absolute risk of dying from smoking (*striped bars*) in all weight categories. (Adapted from Wei M, Kampert JB, Barlow CE, et al: Relationship between low cardiorespiratory fitness and mortality in normal-weight, overweight, and obese men. JAMA 282:1547–1553, 1999.)

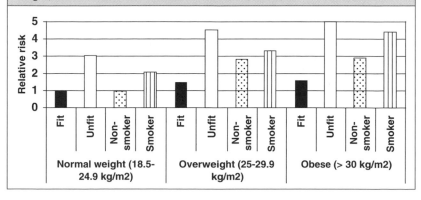

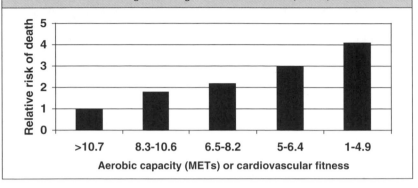

Figure 6–7. The lower the physical fitness (1.0–4.9 METS being the lowest), the greater the relative risk of dying in patients with CVD. (Adapted from Myers J, Prakash M, Froelicher V, et al: Exercise capacity and mortality among men referred for exercise testing. New Engl J Med 346:793–801, 2002.)

Type 2 diabetes:

- Low aerobic fitness and physical inactivity were independent predictors of all-cause mortality in men with type 2 diabetes[20] (Fig 6–8).
- All-cause mortality was greater in men with type 2 diabetes who had low cardiovascular fitness, compared to the men with type 2 diabetes having higher cardiovascular fitness.
- The correlation between low fitness/inactivity and mortality was strong, with adjusted relative risks for death of 2.1 for low fitness and 1.7 for self-reported inactivity.
- Low aerobic fitness (< 5 METs) *triples* the relative risk of dying from

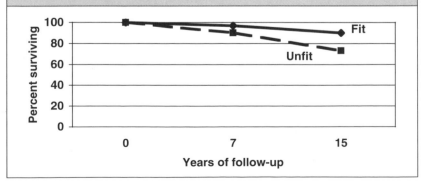

Figure 6–8. In men with type 2 diabetes, physical fitness was an independent predictor of survival. Unfit group = *dashed line,* fit group = *solid line.* (Adapted from Wei M, Gibbons LW, Kampert JB, et al: Low cardiorespiratory fitness and physical inactivity as predictors of mortality in men with type 2 diabetes. Ann Intern Med 132:605–611, 2000.)

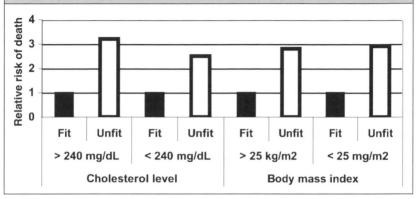

Figure 6–9. An unfit state triples the risk of dying from type 2 diabetes, regardless of cholesterol level or BMI. Low aerobic fitness (< 5 METs) = *white bars*, high aerobic fitness (> 8 METs) = *black bars*. (Adapted from Wei M, Gibbons LW, Kampert JB, et al: Low cardiorespiratory fitness and physical inactivity as predictors of mortality in men with type 2 diabetes. Ann Intern Med 132:605–611, 2000.)

type 2 diabetes regardless of high (> 240 mg/dL) or low (< 240 mg/dL) cholesterol and of high (> 25 kg/m²) or low (< 25 kg/m²) BMI, compared to high aerobic fitness (> 8 METs). See Figure 6–9.

Hypertension, chronic obstructive lung disease, hypercholesterolemia:

- Low aerobic fitness *doubles* the risk of dying in patients with hypertension, chronic obstructive pulmonary disease (COPD), and hypercholesterolemia[17] (Fig 6–10).
- These results were obtained in nondiabetic men.

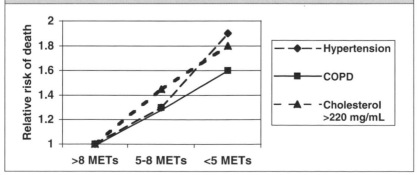

Figure 6–10. In nondiabetic men with hypertension, COPD, and high cholesterol, low cardiovascular fitness (< 5 METS) doubled the risk of dying. (Adapted from Myers J, Prakash M, Froelicher V, et al: Exercise capacity and mortality among men referred for exercise testing. New Engl J Med 346:793–801, 2002.)

TABLE 6–2.	Summary of the Potential Cellular/Biochemical Mechanisms Underlying the Benefits of Physical Activity	
Clinical Manifestation of Physical _In_activity	**Benefits of Increased Daily Physical Activity**	**Potential Cellular/ Biochemical Mechanisms**
Obesity	Reduces total abdominal and visceral adiposity in a dose-response manner	Unknown
Diabetes mellitus, type II	Increases insulin sensitivity of the exercising skeletal muscle and whole body glucose tolerance	Increased translocation of glucose transporter (GLUT4) protein to sarcolemma
Dyslipidemia	Increased clearance of blood total triglycerides, chylomicrons, and VLDL by exercising muscle	Increased gene transcription and protein levels for fatty acid uptake, transfer, oxidation
Atherosclerosis	Increase in luminal diameter of coronary arteries	Nitric oxide inhibits vascular smooth muscle cell pro-liferation, platelet aggregation, monocyte adherence
Hypertension	Regular exercise reduces resting BP and decreases LVH in African-American men with severe hypertension.	Smooth muscle dilatory effects on vascular endothelium mediated by nitric oxide
Vascular	Higher resting and exercise stroke volumes, lower resting and submaximal exercise heart rates, increased capillary density	
Cardiovascular • Angina/MI • Congestive heart failure	Lowers death risk by 20–25% after MI. Improves endothelial function, skeletal muscle aerobic metabolism, stroke volume (via less afterload)	Endothelial-derived nitric oxide produces relaxation of adjacent smooth muscle cells.
Cerebrovascular • Ischemic stroke	Reduction in risk of total and ischemic stroke in a dose-response manner in women	Lowers blood pressure, plasma fibrinogen, platelet aggregation, plasma tPA activity
Peripheral vascular disease • Intermittent claudication	Increases maximal treadmill walking distance by 179 m	Increased vascular relaxation mediated by nitric oxide in blood vessels and increased collateral blood vessels
Pulmonary • Asthma	May reduce development of asthma	Physical training improves cardiopulmonary fitness with-out changing lung function.
• COPD	Dyspnea can be improved despite presence of fixed structural abnormalities in lung	Improved respiratory muscle function, breathing pattern, reduced anxiety

(continued)

TABLE 6–2.   Summary of the Potential Cellular/Biochemical Mechanisms Underlying the Benefits of Physical Activity *(Continued)*

Clinical Manifestation of Physical *In*activity	Benefits of Increased Daily Physical Activity	Potential Cellular/ Biochemical Mechanisms
• Obstructive sleep apnea	Weight loss	Unknown
Malignancy		
• Breast	Decreased risk of breast cancer.	Unknown
• Colon	Decreased risk of colon cancer	Unknown
• Pancreatic	Decreased risk of pancreatic cancer	Unknown
Degenerative conditions		
• Sarcopenia	Resistance training improves muscle strength and size, mobility, spontaneous activity	Mainly improved neural recruitment of existing but underused skeletal muscle with enhanced muscle mass synthesis
• Physical frailty	Postpones disability and enhances independent living even in the oldest-old subjects	Increased muscle strength
• Osteopenia/ osteoporosis	Delays the decrease of bone mineral density	Loading of bone
Infections/immunity		
• HIV/AIDS	Increased cardiopulmonary fitness, CD4 count, psychological status, quality of life	Unknown; however, moderate exercise improves immune system while intense exercise suppresses it.
Musculoskeletal		
• Rheumatoid arthritis	Regular exercise does not exacerbate pain or accelerate disease progression.	Unknown
• Low back pain	Helps chronic low back pain patients to increase return to normal daily activities and work	Unknown
Neurologic	Running enhances neurogenesis, water maze performance, and long-term potentiation.	Exercise induces brain IGF-I, which mediates protective effects by enhancing cerebellar angiogenesis, hippocampal survival of newborn cells, brain norepinephrine, serotonin, brain-derived neurotrophic factor, FGF-2 levels
• Alzheimer's disease	Women with higher levels of baseline physical activity are less likely to develop cognitive decline.	Unknown

(continued)

TABLE 6–2. Summary of the Potential Cellular/Biochemical Mechanisms Underlying the Benefits of Physical Activity *(Continued)*		
Clinical Manifestation of Physical *In*activity	**Benefits of Increased Daily Physical Activity**	**Potential Cellular/ Biochemical Mechanisms**
• Multiple sclerosis	Improved functional performance, quality of life, fatigue associated with disease	Unknown
Recovery after surgery/ immobilization/injury/ debilitating illnesses	Decreases morbidity, mortality, rehospitalizations while improving quality of life, depression scores, physical functioning	Unknown
Smoking cessation	Exercise training as a sole intervention does not appear to enhance smoking cessation.	Unknown
Psychiatric/psychologic		
• Depression	Antidepressant and anxiolytic effects	Unknown
Gallstones	Decreased risk of chole- cystectomy independent of other risk factors for gallstone disease, such as obesity	Improves glucose tolerance, blood lipid levels, cholecystokinin release while reducing estrogen exposure

BP = blood pressure, FGF2 = fibroblast growth factor 2, GLUT4 = glucose transporter 4, IGF-I = insulin-like growth factor–I, LVH = left ventricular hypertrophy, MI = myocardial infarction, tPA = tissue plasminogen activator, VLDL = very low density lipoproteins
Data from Chakravarthy MV, Joyner MJ, Booth FW: An obligation for primary care physicians to prescribe physical activity to sedentary patients to reduce the risk of chronic health conditions. Mayo Clin Proc 77:165–173, 2002.

Summary of the Health Benefits of Physical Activity

Low maximal aerobic capacity, i.e., low cardiovascular fitness, is associated with decreased survival (or increased relative risk of death) in healthy persons and patients with the following chronic health conditions (CHCs):

Cardiovascular disease
Chronic obstructive lung disease
Type 2 diabetes
Hypercholesterolemia
Hypertension
Smoking
Obesity

The magnitude of the effects of low cardiovascular fitness on mortality is great, usually being two-fold or more between low and high cardiovascular fitness. Therefore, primary prevention with increased physical activity would delay the decline in cardiovascular fitness that occurs with physical inactivity and aging. No single drug presently exists that could have such a potent beneficial effect on the primary prevention of CHCs. Increasing physical activity would thus have a tremendous public health benefit by decreasing mortality. Physical activity remains one of the most efficacious preventive therapeutic modalities to protect against CHCs.

Suggested Reading

1. Lichtenstein P, Holm NV, Verkasalo PK, et al. Environmental and heritable factors in the causation of cancer—Analyses of cohorts of twins from Sweden, Denmark, and Finland. N Engl J Med 343:78–85, 2000.
2. Hu FB, Manson JE, Stampfer MJ, et al. Diet, lifestyle, and the risk of type 2 diabetes mellitus in women. N Engl J Med 345: 790–797, 2001.
3. Stampfer MJ, Hu FB, Manson JE, Rimm EB, Willett WC. Primary prevention of coronary heart disease in women through diet and lifestyle. N Engl J Med. 343:16–22, 2000.
4. Martinez ME, Giovannucci E, Spiegelman D, et al. Leisure-time physical activity, body size, and colon cancer in women. Nurses' Health Study Research Group. J Natl Cancer Inst 89:948–955, 1997.
5. Rockhill B, Willett WC, Manson JE, et al. Physical activity and mortality: A prospective study among women. Am J Public Health 91:578–583, 2001.
6. Rockhill B, Willett WC, Hunter DJ, et al. A prospective study of recreational physical activity and breast cancer risk. Arch Intern Med 159:2290–2296, 1999.
7. Pate RR, Pratt M, Blair SN, et al. Physical activity and public health. A recommendation from the Centers for Disease Control and Prevention and the American College of Sports Medicine. JAMA 273:402–407, 1995.
8. Reference deleted.
9. Fletcher GF, Balady G, Blair SN, et al. Statement on exercise: Benefits and recommendations for physical activity programs for all Americans. A statement for health professionals by the Committee on Exercise and Cardiac Rehabilitation of the Council on Clinical Cardiology, American Heart Association. Circulation 94:857–62, 1996.
10. Kesaniemi YK, Danforth E Jr, Jensen MD, et al. Dose-response issues concerning physical activity and health: An evidence-based symposium. Med Sci Sports Exerc 33(6 Suppl): S351–58, 2001.
11. Mokdad AH, Bowman BA, Ford ES, et al. The continuing epidemics of obesity and diabetes in the United States. JAMA 286: 1195–1200, 2001.
12. Hu FB, Sigal RJ, Rich-Edwards JW, et al. Walking compared with vigorous physical activity and risk of type 2 diabetes in women: A prospective study. JAMA 282: 1433–1439, 1999.
13. Hu FB, Stampfer MJ, Colditz GA, et al. Physical activity and risk of stroke in women. JAMA 283: 2961–2967, 2000.
14. Manson JE, Hu FB, Rich-Edwards JW, et al. A prospective study of walking as compared with vigorous exercise in the prevention of coronary heart disease in women. New Engl J Med 341: 650–658, 1999.

15. Knowler WC, Barrett-Connor E, Fowler SE, et al. Reduction in the incidence of type 2 diabetes with lifestyle intervention or metformin. New Engl J Med 346:393–403, 2002.
16. Tuomilehto J, Lindstrom J, Eriksson JG, et al. Prevention of type 2 diabetes mellitus by changes in lifestyle among subjects with impaired glucose tolerance. New Engl J Med 344:1343–1350, 2001.
17. Myers J, Prakash M, Froelicher V, et al. Exercise capacity and mortality among men referred for exercise testing. N Engl J Med 346:793–801, 2002.
18. Blair SN, Kohl HW III, et al. Changes in physical fitness and all-cause mortality. A prospective study of healthy and unhealthy men. JAMA 273(14):1093–1098, 1995.
19. Wei M, Kampert JB, Barlow CE, et al. Relationship between low cardiorespiratory fitness and mortality in normal-weight, overweight, and obese men. JAMA 282:1547–1553, 1999.
20. Wei M, Gibbons LW, Kampert JB, Nichaman MZ, Blair SN. Low cardiorespiratory fitness and physical inactivity as predictors of mortality in men with type 2 diabetes. Ann Intern Med. 132:605–611, 2000.
21. Chakravarthy MV, Joyner MJ, Booth FW. An obligation for primary care physicians to prescribe physical activity to sedentary patients to reduce the risk of chronic health conditions. Mayo Clin Proc 77:165–173, 2002.

Caloric Balance and Expenditure

chapter

7

Caloric Expenditures

The number of calories expended each day can be divided into two categories: fixed and variable. **Fixed** caloric expenditure occurs via resting metabolic rate (minimal physiological activities while awake or asleep) and digestion of food. There is little external manipulation of this number. **Variable** caloric expenditure is subject to changing physical activity levels.

Quantification of Work

Work = Force × Distance Moved

A common unit employed to measure heat energy is the kilocalorie (kcal). One kcal is the amount of heat required to raise the temperature of 1 kg of water by 1° C. To convert kcals to standard international (SI) units: 1 kcal = 4186 joules. We use the term calorie here because American food containers list calories, not joules. The term kcal in this book refers to caloric expenditure, because it allows us to teach the concept of caloric balance—the key to body fat content. We use the words calorie and kilocalorie interchangeably, because food containers print the term "kilocalorie" as "calorie," while the exact scientific expression is "kilocalorie."

Language of Caloric Expenditure

Absolute intensity of voluntary physical activity is the number of calories expended. Its units can be calories/min or kilocalories/min. To convert kilocalories to metabolic equivalent of the task (MET): the number of kilocalories expended at rest = 1 MET (i.e., metabolic rate). MET is an index of the actual rate of caloric expenditure and can be used to prescribe exercise intensity for patients.

Maximal caloric expenditure occurs when the body can no longer increase its caloric expenditure as the intensity of exercise increases.

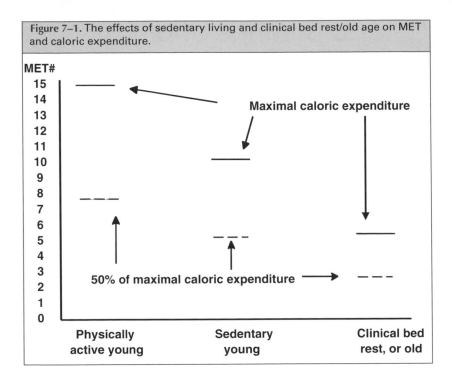

Figure 7–1. The effects of sedentary living and clinical bed rest/old age on MET and caloric expenditure.

Maximal caloric expenditure can be expressed in units of maximal kcal/min, i.e., maximal oxygen consumed by the body/min. It decreases with aging and with physical inactivity (Fig. 7–1).

The concept of absolute work intensity is important in physical activity prescription because:

- The higher the work intensity (moving from light to heavy work), the shorter the time of work duration until fatigue occurs.
- A certain number of METs must be spent in physical activity each week in order to pass a "health threshold." Though the minimal effective dose is not well defined, physical activity exceeding 1000 kcal/wk (4200 kJ/wk) has been associated with a 30% reduction in all-cause mortality rates. However, any health threshold varies among individuals and for specific chronic health conditions dependent upon polymorphisms in disease-susceptible genes.
- MET values for various work tasks allow physicians to match prescribed MET values to specific activities (see Appendix I).
- Injury rate increases as exercise intensity (MET) increases.
- Patient compliance may decrease as exercise intensity (MET) increases.

How Caloric Imbalance Increases Body Fat

Caloric balance simply means:

kilocalories in = kilocalories out.

Estimating "calories in" is easier than estimating "calories out." Since exact estimates of caloric expenditure outside of a research lab are impossible, discussions of weight-control focus on calories eaten. However, individuals eating many calories are not necessarily overweight, because physical activity can mitigate the effects of their caloric imbalance. As an example, consider lumberjacks who use manual labor (not power saws) to cut trees, eat 4500–8000 calories per day, and are very muscular, with low percentages of body fat. They do not gain body fat because their voluntary caloric expenditure allows their net caloric balance to be zero (6000 calories in minus 6000 calories out = zero change in body fat).

A relatively small positive caloric imbalance (i.e., calories in > calories out) each day translates to excess fat (Fig. 7–2 and 7–3). A positive caloric imbalance of only 10 kilocalories each day for 365 days equates to the caloric equivalent of 1 pound of fat at the end of 1 year:

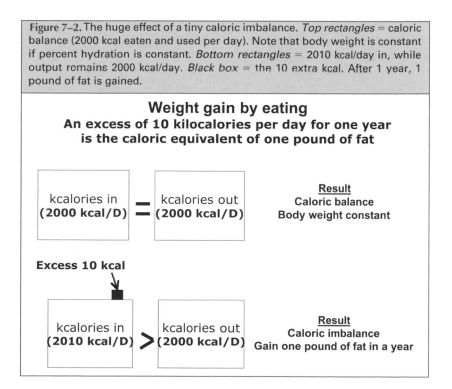

Figure 7–2. The huge effect of a tiny caloric imbalance. *Top rectangles* = caloric balance (2000 kcal eaten and used per day). Note that body weight is constant if percent hydration is constant. *Bottom rectangles* = 2010 kcal/day in, while output remains 2000 kcal/day. *Black box* = the 10 extra kcal. After 1 year, 1 pound of fat is gained.

Weight gain by eating
An excess of 10 kilocalories per day for one year
is the caloric equivalent of one pound of fat

| kcalories in (2000 kcal/D) | — | kcalories out (2000 kcal/D) | Result Caloric balance Body weight constant |

Excess 10 kcal

| kcalories in (2010 kcal/D) | > | kcalories out (2000 kcal/D) | Result Caloric imbalance Gain one pound of fat in a year |

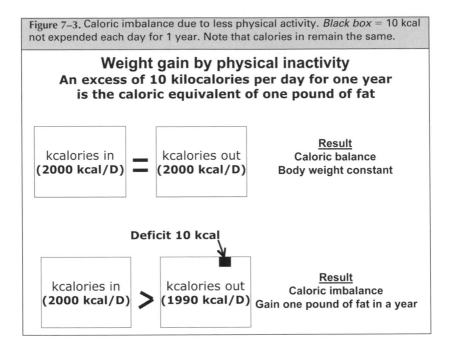

Figure 7–3. Caloric imbalance due to less physical activity. *Black box* = 10 kcal not expended each day for 1 year. Note that calories in remain the same.

- 10 positive calories over caloric balance × 365 days per year = 3650 positive calories per year
- 1 pound of fat = ~3500 kilocalories
- 1 pound of fat per year × 20 years (from age of 20 to 40 years) = 20 pounds of fat gained in 20 years, which is what many middle-aged Americans gain!

Simply put, a positive caloric imbalance is the result of eating too much and/or moving around (exercising) too little. Figures 7–2 and 7–3 demonstrate that overnutrition and physical inactivity are *equivalent calorically* in the production of 1 pound of fat.

Key Points: Fat Gain

∞ Gaining body fat requires only a small positive caloric imbalance.

∞ Primary prevention for body fat gain thus requires only a small adjustment down in caloric intake, or a small adjustment up in caloric expenditure (via physical activity).

∞ Primary prevention of weight gain needs to be especially emphasized for those patients who have a chart history of increasing BMI from 20 to 25 kg/m².

Healthcare professionals should educate their patients about caloric balance and should actively counsel them to drop one energy-dense food, or increase physical activity to expend an additional 10 kcal/day. (See Chapters 8–10 for specific details on counseling patients about these topics.) Have your office staff call patients with weight problems every 6 months to check on body weight. Institute early interventions if BMI continues to rise (before BMI exceeds 26 kg/m^2).

Biological Basis of Losing Body Fat

Though it seems to follow logically, a 10 kcal deficit per day over the course of a year does *not* extrapolate to a loss of 1 pound of body fat. This is a very important concept. Caloric deficits *much greater than* 10 kcal each day must occur to cause the loss of 1 pound of fat after 1 year. Healthcare professionals prescribing weight loss must advise daily caloric deficits of 500 calories or more. The explanation for this is fascinating: we inherited a genetic trait from our ancestors that defends against losses in body weight. In 10,000 B.C., survival literally depended on the ability to efficiently conserve fat. Those individuals who survived are speculated to have had "thrifty genes" that more efficiently stored fat in times of feast and then more efficiently used this fat during famine portions of the life cycle (Fig 7–4). Thus, we are programmed to efficiently store fat in periods of "feasting." Since in the 21st century we

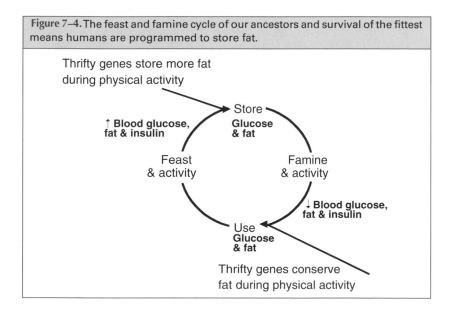

Figure 7–4. The feast and famine cycle of our ancestors and survival of the fittest means humans are programmed to store fat.

Thrifty genes store more fat during physical activity

↑ Blood glucose, fat & insulin

Store Glucose & fat

Feast & activity

Famine & activity

↓ Blood glucose, fat & insulin

Use Glucose & fat

Thrifty genes conserve fat during physical activity

are in a state of continuous "feast," concomitant with a drastic decline in physical activity/labor, it is that much harder to overcome our genetically predisposed need to store fat. This is why our bodies require greater caloric deficits to "take off" a pound of fat than to "put on" a pound of fat (Fig. 7–5).

One potential biological explanation was provided by Liebel et al, who reported that when losing body weight through dieting, resting metabolism fell to conserve the body weight during the period of reduced caloric intake.[1] However, others contend that the lower resting metabolism is proportional to the loss in body mass. For example, Wing and Hill have not been able to document a clear metabolic state consistent with the notion of increased "metabolic efficiency" in obese subjects attempting to lose body fat.[2]

As efficiency of defending against a drop in body weight varies between individuals (remember that some people's genes are more "thrifty" than others), precise quantification of the negative caloric imbalance (i.e., the size of the caloric deficit) needed by the patient each day to lose 1 pound of fat is unknown. Wing and Hill's review concluded that physical activity goals for weight management programs may need to be substantially higher than those for the general population[2] (Fig. 7–6). They state that healthcare professionals do not have a good database with

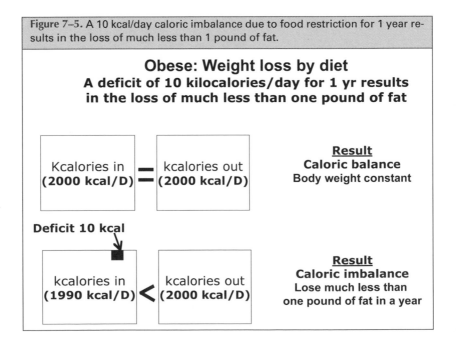

Figure 7–5. A 10 kcal/day caloric imbalance due to food restriction for 1 year results in the loss of much less than 1 pound of fat.

Obese: Weight loss by diet
A deficit of 10 kilocalories/day for 1 yr results in the loss of much less than one pound of fat

| Kcalories in (2000 kcal/D) | **—** | kcalories out (2000 kcal/D) | **Result** Caloric balance Body weight constant |

Deficit 10 kcal

| kcalories in (1990 kcal/D) | **<** | kcalories out (2000 kcal/D) | **Result** Caloric imbalance Lose much less than one pound of fat in a year |

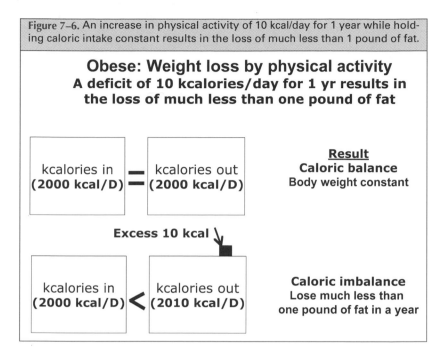

Figure 7–6. An increase in physical activity of 10 kcal/day for 1 year while holding caloric intake constant results in the loss of much less than 1 pound of fat.

which to develop specific physical activity guidelines to prevent weight gain—and that developing such a database should be a high priority. The Institute of Medicine has just concluded that at least 1 hour of moderate-intensity physical activity by adults each day is required to prevent weight gain and accrue additional, weight-independent benefits.

Key Points: Weight Loss

- Healthcare professionals must prescribe caloric deficits of at least 500 kcal/day or more to institute a loss of ≥ 1 lb of fat per year.
- However, reducing the caloric balance by only 10 kcal/day for 1 year *is* sufficient to *prevent* a gain of 1 pound of fat.
- Given that prevention of the gain in 1 pound of fat in 1 year follows the 10 kcal/day rule, it becomes quite obvious that primary prevention is easier than weight loss!

Physical Activity As Primary Prevention

In children and adolescents, small increases in moderate daily physical activity prevent large increases in body fat, as long as caloric intake does not increase to compensate for the increased physical activity.

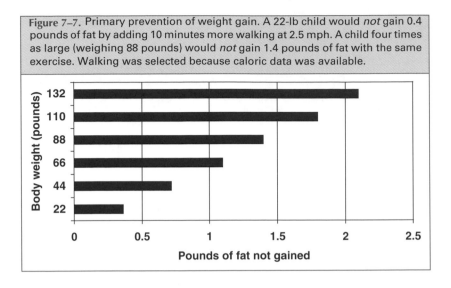

Figure 7-7. Primary prevention of weight gain. A 22-lb child would *not* gain 0.4 pounds of fat by adding 10 minutes more walking at 2.5 mph. A child four times as large (weighing 88 pounds) would *not* gain 1.4 pounds of fat with the same exercise. Walking was selected because caloric data was available.

Adding 10 minutes of walking per day at a speed of 2.5 mph for 1 year without any other changes can prevent body fat gain by children/ adolescents of various body weights (Fig 7-7). As body weight determines caloric expenditure, the same distance walked by smaller children would prevent gaining fewer pounds of fat than a larger child. Therefore, replacement of sedentary time (such as TV watching) with physical activity is an important primary prevention modality for pediatric obesity.

Television Equivalents

An 88-pound child/adolescent substituting 1 hour of TV with 30 min of walking and 30 min of other sedentary activity (other than TV, such as reading) for 1 year would *not* gain 4.5 lbs of fat (Fig. 7-8). Remarkably, the same substitutions in a 220-lb child/adolescent would prevent the gain of *11 pounds of fat in a year!*

The concept of TV equivalents only works in the *prevention* of gain in body fat; it does not work in the *loss* of body fat. Unfortunately the principles of caloric balance for the prevention of a gain in body fat by the expenditure of calories in physical activity do not extend to a loss in body fat because the body adapts to its newer, greater body weight and then defends against weight loss. Thus, primary prevention to avoid body fat gain in the first place requires fewer calories expended as physical activity, than does tertiary prevention to remove the already added/stored body fat.

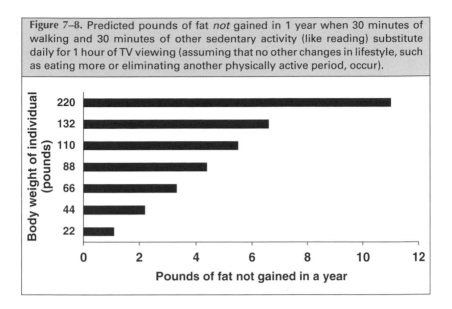

Figure 7–8. Predicted pounds of fat *not* gained in 1 year when 30 minutes of walking and 30 minutes of other sedentary activity (like reading) substitute daily for 1 hour of TV viewing (assuming that no other changes in lifestyle, such as eating more or eliminating another physically active period, occur).

The question is, would substitution of physical activity for 1 hour of TV viewing each day be enough to prevent pediatric obesity? We believe the answer is "Yes."

Fat gain prevented as a child ages from 7 to 17 years:

- Using the CDC tables for age-BMI (see Figs. 10–8 and 10–9 in Chapter 10), a 7-year-old boy weighing 59.4 lbs who remains in the 85th percentile of body weight would weigh 173.8 lbs (85th percentile) 10 yrs later at age 17. However, if the same adolescent weighed 195.8 lbs (95th percentile) at age 17, then 22 lbs (difference between the 85th and 95th percentiles) of extra weight would have to be accumulated during growth between ages 7 and 17.
- Thus, the primary prevention goal in this patient would be to prevent gaining 22 lbs of fat from the age of 7 to 17 years (an average of 2.2 lbs/yr). Note that moving from the 84th percentile to the 86th percentile crosses from the "normal" body weight category to the "overweight" category (the 85th percentile is the threshold line to enter the pediatric overweight category).

Physical activity required to prevent gaining 1 pound of fat:

- Children expend a net of 1 kcal/2.2 pounds of body weight/mile walked, whereas adolescents use 0.9 kcal/2.2 pounds/mile walked.
- 10 kcal needs to be expended every day for 365 days to equate to about 1 lb of fat.

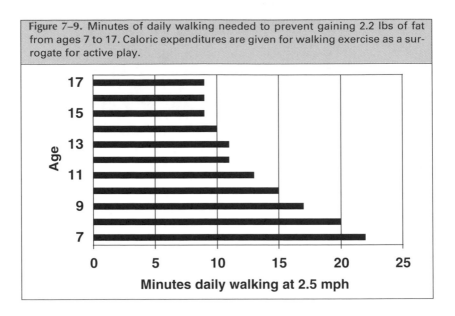

Figure 7–9. Minutes of daily walking needed to prevent gaining 2.2 lbs of fat from ages 7 to 17. Caloric expenditures are given for walking exercise as a surrogate for active play.

Physical activity required to prevent gaining 22 pounds of fat from the ages of 7 to 17, or gaining 2.2 lbs of fat per year:

- The amount of walking needed to prevent a gain of 2.2 pounds of fat each year from the ages of 7 to 17 decreases from 22 min/day to 8 min/day[3,4] (Fig. 7–9).
- The explanation is that body weight increases with age, and the greater the body weight, the greater the number of calories expended walking. The caloric cost is greater for moving a heavier object than a light object, as work = force × distance, where force = mass × acceleration. As body mass increases, greater caloric expenditure occurs, and fewer minutes of walking are needed to expend calories.

Summary: Primary Prevention of Pediatric Obesity

It is not unreasonable to ask a child to replace one sedentary event with walking/active play. This is an achievable goal that will prevent the gain of too much fat during the growing period. The science predicts that substituting physical activity (such as moderate walking) for a sedentary event (such as TV viewing) significantly contributes to a reduction in body fat gain.

If the physical activity were to be more vigorous than walking, then fewer minutes would be needed each day to consume the number of calories required to prevent the gain of 22 pounds of fat in the 10-yr-period (see Fig. 7–9). One additional confounding variable in these calculations is that children become more sedentary as they age. Indeed, the evolution of sedentary habits while growing up is likely a major contributor to the gain of body fat. Thus, the number of minutes of physical activity at any given age is for illustration only, as the child will not present with a quantitative record of current daily physical activity upon which to prescribe a quantitative increase in physical activity. Rather, prescription of increased physical activity will have to be qualitative.

Prescribing increased physical activity is most effective for the *prevention of a gain* in body fat, as the body defends itself against a loss in body fat by unknown mechanisms. However, the body does *not* lower resting metabolism when physical activity is increased to prevent a weight gain. Thus, it is common sense to prevent gain in body fat, rather than try to lose fat once already gained.

Suggested Reading

1. Leibel RL, Rosenbaum M, Hirsch J. Changes in energy expenditure resulting from altered body weight. N Engl J Med 332:621–628, 1995.
2. Wing RR, Hill JO. Successful weight loss maintenance. Ann Rev Nutr 21:323–41, 2001.
3. Walker JL, Murray TD, Jackson AS, et al. The energy cost of horizontal walking and running in adolescents. Med Sci Sports Exerc 31:311–322, 1999.
4. McCann DJ, Adams WC. A dimensional paradigm for identifying the size-independent cost of walking. Med Sci Sports Exerc 34:1009–1017, 2002.

Physical Activity Prescription

chapter

8

It is difficult to convince physicians to institute programs of physical activity for their sedentary patients. Prescriptions and counseling require constant attention and assessment, and a simple "go and exercise" message to patients is not sufficient. However, since there is overwhelming evidence that it is possible to reduce heart disease, stroke, and type 2 diabetes incidence by ~30% by engaging in ≥ 3 hours/week of moderate-intensity physical activity, the effort is certainly worthwhile. This amount of physical exercise per week can be accumulated easily, by engaging in both unstructured/unsupervised and structured/supervised activities.

Furthermore, the health benefits can be accrued without weight loss. Unfortunately, as Bouxsein and Marcus stated: " . . . exercise is not a way of life for most adults. Men and women commonly assert that regular exercise is not necessary at their age; they frequently have unrealistic expectations regarding the health benefits of their daily activities, and they seriously exaggerate the risks of vigorous exercise. Exercise strategies for the general population must be simple and flexible to accommodate individuals with average motivation, limited access to equipment, and busy schedules."[1]

Given the tremendous benefits of undertaking routine physical activity in our daily lives, it follows that our healthcare professionals should be trained in the basics of exercise prescription for health-related and quality-of-life benefits.

General Principles of Physical Activity Prescription

Key Elements of Physical Activity Prescription Programs

Screening for sedentary lifestyle when taking a history and performing a physical exam should be just as routine as screening for smoking and checking family history, blood pressure, lipids, blood glucose, etc. Moreover, a physical activity prescription should be included with other heathcare recommendations, and should be managed just as seriously and with the same diligence that accompanies prescribing antibiotics or other medications. Consider, too, that many individuals have no insurance, nor the monies to pay for even basic medications, and a prescription for physical activity can be an effective alternative to expensive drugs in many conditions.

A physical activity prescription should be:

- Given in a concise and specific manner in terms of the modality, frequency, intensity, and duration (see sample plans on following pages).
- Accompanied by advice regarding safety, practical ideas for implementation, and behavioral support systems for monitoring progress and providing feedback.
- Used as a preventive medicine modality, similar to the concept of recommending smoking cessation for reducing cardiovascular risks.

Proper documentation is required for effective assessment, monitoring of progress, and conveyance of meaningful follow-up comments. Documentation can be facilitated by use of simple forms or flow charts (see Appendix II for an example.)

The Dosage of Physical Activity

The amount of physical inactivity required to exceed a threshold of biological significance to produce an overt clinical disease varies with the individual. For patients with a family history of a chronic disease, it is important to prescribe *some* degree of physical activity, as much as their present condition can tolerate.

Consensus reports have commonly recommended moderate exercise (e.g., brisk walking) for individuals who are currently sedentary, rather than hard physical activity (e.g., running or working out at > 60% of aerobic capacity, or > 6 METS). Small increases in physical activity in completely sedentary individuals have been shown to have significant impact on the prevention of many chronic health conditions.

Analogous to the importance of prescribing the correct dose of a medication, it is just as necessary to prescribe the appropriate "dose" of physical activity. Too little of the drug has insufficient efficacy; too much of it has adverse side effects. Similarly, too little physical activity is not effective, and too much may produce negative side effects such as injury (e.g., overuse injuries, which are due to exercising at levels inappropriate for an individual's conditioning). Unfortunately, prescribing physical activity is much more complex and less exact than prescribing a medication. The proper dosage of activity is based on two important concepts: threshold and dose-response effect.

- An **activity threshold** (threshold = the minimum dose necessary to produce an effect) must be achieved to obtain health benefits for various diseases (Fig. 8–1 and Table 8–1).

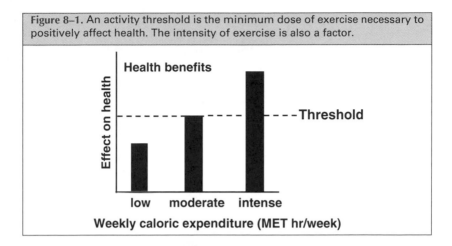

Figure 8–1. An activity threshold is the minimum dose of exercise necessary to positively affect health. The intensity of exercise is also a factor.

Table 8–1. Evidence for Physical Activity Dose-Response Effect and MET Quantification in the Prevention of Increased Morbidity and Mortality from Chronic Health Conditions[2–4]

Disorder	Activity Threshold Needed for Preventive Effects	Effects	Dose-Response for Preventive Effects	Evidence Category*
All-cause mortality	1000 kcal/wk	Lowers mortality	Yes	C
Cardiovascular disease				
Coronary heart disease	4–6 METS/min	Lowers prevalence	Yes	C
Atherosclerosis	1500 kcal/wk	Retardation of progression	Yes	C
	> 2000 kcal/wk	Regression of plaques		
Hypertension	3–5 times/wk during sessions of 30–60 min at an intensity of 40–70% maximal exercise performance	Systolic and diastolic pressures reduced by 7.7 and 5.8 mmHg, respectively	No. Further increases in exercise intensity do not have additional effect	A and B
Cancer				
Breast cancer	4hr/wk at 4–5 MET or 24.5 MET-hrs/wk of vigorous activity	Lowers prevalence	Yes	C
Colon cancer	1000 kcal/wk	Lowers prevalence	Yes	C
Diabetes type 2 (in patients with glucose intolerance)	Unknown	Lowers prevalence	Yes	A

(continued)

Table 8–1. Evidence for Physical Activity Dose-Response Effect and MET Quantification in the Prevention of Increased Morbidity and Mortality from Chronic Health Conditions[2–4] (Continued)

Disorder	Activity Threshold Needed for Preventive Effects	Effects	Dose-Response for Preventive Effects	Evidence Category*
Ischemic stroke	A potential U-shape relationship	Lowers prevalence	Lowers risk at moderate intensity, but no change in inactive or high-intensity activity	C
Lipids				
HDL-cholesterol	1000–1200 kcal/wk	HDL-C is increased by 4.6%	Unknown	B
Triglycerides	Low	Transient decrease occurs 18–24 hrs post exercise	Total exercise volume, not intensity, is more critical. Greater the total volume, lower the blood triglycerides	B and C
Obesity				
Prevention of weight gain	2100–2800 kcal/wk	Loss of weight (avg >60 lbs), and kept it off > 6 years	Yes	C
Osteoporosis	Unknown	Lower prevalence	Both intensity and volume of exercise important	B
Platelet adhesiveness and aggregation	Unknown	Decreased adhesion and aggregation	Unknown	B

*Evidence Categories:
A—Evidence from endpoints of well-designed, randomized clinical trial (RCT) that provide a consistent pattern of findings. Requires substantial numbers of studies, each involving a substantial number of participants.
B—Evidence is from endpoints of intervention that include only a limited number of RCTs, post hoc or subgroup analysis of RCTs, or meta-analysis of RCTs. Pertains when few randomized trials exist; they are small; and the trial results are somewhat inconsistent.
C—Evidence is from outcomes of uncontrolled or nonrandomized trials or from observational studies.

- A **dose-response effect** applies to physical activity. There are proportional changes between intensity (type and duration of exercise) and effect (health benefits).

While there are epidemiological reports demonstrating that mortality reduction and chronic disease prevention can result from achieving the exercise threshold and the ideal dose-response effect, it is unclear whether increasing intensity of physical activity would yield greater benefits in the *treatment* of chronic disease. Also, a subpopulation of patients appears not to have an exercise threshold and is not affected by a dose-response relationship. For example, some patients who exercise at moderate intensity for 30 min/day would still show no increase in their plasma HDL cholesterol concentrations, whereas in an average individual, there is a threshold effect on this parameter. This probably can be explained by presence of individual polymorphisms of specific genes.

Composition of a Physical Activity Plan

Most effective training regimens are a combination of: (1) strength/power, (2) speed and aerobic endurance, and (3) flexibility (Fig. 8–2).[5] We contend that to implement a training regimen, these components must become a part of our daily routines.

Lifestyle modification: Individualizing an exercise plan allows adoption of changes consistent with a person's life circumstances, cultural attitudes, and environment, with the goal of finding opportunities within daily routines to reduce sedentary behavior.

Strength: Muscle strength is built by a muscle group generating force against resistance. A single set of 8–12 repetitions using 8–10 different exercise sets, performed two to three times per week, is sufficient. Each repetition should be performed slowly through a full range of motion without holding the breath (exhale during the lift for 2–4 sec and inhale during lowering of the weight for 4–6 sec). The training should involve

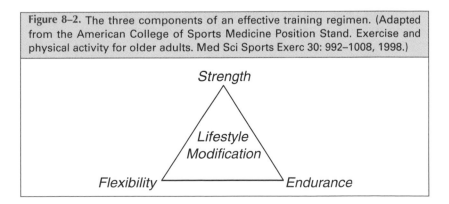

Figure 8–2. The three components of an effective training regimen. (Adapted from the American College of Sports Medicine Position Stand. Exercise and physical activity for older adults. Med Sci Sports Exerc 30: 992–1008, 1998.)

Strength

Lifestyle Modification

Flexibility   *Endurance*

all clinically relevant muscle groups (hip extensors, knee extensors, ankle plantar flexors and dorsiflexors, biceps, triceps, shoulders, back extensors, and abdominal muscles)

Endurance: Aerobic exercise is activity that results in an increased heart rate for an extended period of time. It improves stamina and cardiopulmonary fitness. The goal is moderate aerobic activity for a cumulative total of at least 30 min, most days of the week, with individual bouts of activity being as brief as 10 min in duration. *Light activity* is < 4 METs; *moderate activity* is 4–6 METs (corresponds to walking on level ground at a 4.0–4.5 mph pace, i.e. brisk walk); *heavy activity* is > 6 METs (see Appendix I for further details of MET quantification and corresponding examples of daily activities).

Flexibility: Major muscle groups should be stretched once per day after exercise, when muscles are more compliant, and should be done in a "stretch and hold" fashion, avoiding "ballistic" or "bouncing" stretches.

The performance of all three of these modalities *daily* by sedentary individuals is somewhat unrealistic. They should be spread over the course of the whole week, arriving at a total average of 3.5–4.0 hours per week. It is indeed difficult to incorporate more physical activity into already packed daily routines, and perhaps the focus should be on establishing a routine of some kind, especially in those individuals who are completely sedentary. But also note that this time commitment—to enhancing and enriching one's health—is merely one-sixth of the average adult's weekly discretional leisure time! Moreover, there are cost-benefits of a healthy lifestyle. Finally, educate your patients that such a lifestyle is truly effective in both preventing and managing chronic diseases. Encourage them to seek professional guidance from programs such as INTERVENT (http://www.interventusa.com) and WellCoaches (http://www.wellcoaches.com), as well as from local experts at wellness/fitness centers.

Completely sedentary patients should initiate activity at a very low level; graded increments can be added gradually to reach a goal of moderate activity (defined using heart rate and VO_2 max ranges, rating of perceived exertion, and MET charts for specific activities; see Appendix 1). For the sake of simplicity, patients should exercise at the maximal intensity at which they are still able to carry on a conversation comfortably (the "talk test"). Similarly, for resistance exercises, previously completely sedentary patients should begin slowly and gradually advance the intensity of their training regimen (by starting with resistive bands/tubing and light weights of ~2 lbs). However, to gain strength and prevent the long-term loss of previous strength gains, training needs to be progressively more intense with increasing weight lifted.

For *all* individuals, warm-up and cool-down periods consisting of 5–10 min of less-intense activity (e.g., slow walking, stretching) are important to decrease the risk of hypotension and musculoskeletal or cardiovascular complications.

A physical activity plan is a dynamic process. It should be structured to accommodate an individual patient's current goals and needs, take into full account any pre-existing comorbidities, and be responsive to changes over time. In the spirit of the oath to do no harm to your patients, you might suggest—if there are no health concerns related to brisk walking or stair climbing—that sedentary patients begin modifying their lifestyle to incorporate these activities. Exceptions do exist; see later in this chapter for details regarding the identification of high-risk patients, risk stratification, and contraindications to physical activity prescription.

Designing Appropriate Physical Activity Programs for Sedentary Individuals

It is unrealistic to expect patients, especially completely sedentary patients to instantaneously begin engaging in 30 min/day of moderate physical activity. Approximately 25% of the U.S. population (40% in some subgroups) was completely sedentary in 1995. It is reasonable to speculate that this number has significantly increased since then. Therefore, we need to investigate and employ alternative strategies to convince completely sedentary individuals to become more physically active.

A potential approach includes a combination of structured and/or unstructured programs (Fig. 8–3). In both forms of physical activity, encourage the use of pedometers to track lifestyle activity, such as incorporating 10,000 steps/day for cardiovascular fitness and 14,000 steps/day for weight loss management. See http://www.digiwalker.com for more details. Interestingly, unstructured (i.e., lifestyle) physical activity programs were as effective as structured exercise programs, as shown by the ACTIVE trial.[6]

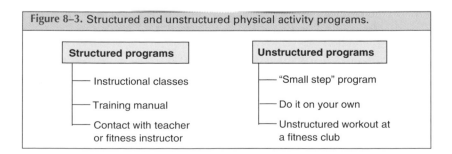

Figure 8–3. Structured and unstructured physical activity programs.

Structured programs	Unstructured programs
— Instructional classes	— "Small step" program
— Training manual	— Do it on your own
— Contact with teacher or fitness instructor	— Unstructured workout at a fitness club

Project ACTIVE: A Comparison of Structured and Unstructured Physical Activity[6]

Experimental design: 235 healthy sedentary men (n = 116) and women (n = 119) aged 35 to 60 years were randomized to either a lifestyle (unstructured) physical activity program or a structured exercise program. Exclusion criteria were—

- Self-reported history of myocardial infarction, stroke, type 1 diabetes mellitus, osteoporosis, and osteoarthritis (if it limited mobility)
- Weight more than 140% of ideal body weight
- Three or more drinks of alcohol daily
- Exercising at least 3 days a week for ≥ 20 minutes or having an estimated total energy expenditure exceeding 36 kcal/kg per day (men) or 34 kcal/kg per day (women)
- Blood pressure of ≥ 160/100 mmHg
- Use of medication (such as beta-blockers) that could impair exercise performance
- For women, plans to become pregnant in the next 2 years.

Results: A lifestyle physical activity intervention was as effective as a structured exercise program, and was more cost-effective than a structured program in improving physical activity and cardiorespiratory health. Effectiveness was measured by—

- Increasing energy expenditure by 1%
- Reducing body fat by 2%
- Reducing systolic (4%) and diastolic (5%) blood pressures
- Increasing peak oxygen uptake by 1%.

The average clinical changes for all subjects may seem small, but one-fifth of initially sedentary participants were achieving or exceeding public health recommendations for 30 minutes of physical activity at the end of 24 months. One-quarter of subjects had maintained an increase in cardiorespiratory fitness of 10% or more at the end of 24 months. The 10% increase in treadmill performance in the Project ACTIVE study might result in a 15% reduction in all-cause mortality. Indeed, increasing fitness levels (for example, in those with VO_2 max > 2.2 L/min compared to those with < 1.5 L/min) reduced risk of CAD mortality by ~60%. Increasing physical activity in CAD patients also markedly reduced the risk for recurrent cardiac events.

These results have convinced us that prescribing *unstructured* programs may be a more effective way to encourage sedentary individuals, as well as a particular subset of the population (Table 8–2), to engage in regular physical activity within the framework of their daily routines.

Table 8–2. A Subset of the Population That May Benefit From Unstructured Exercise Programs
Individuals who do NOT have:
• Health insurance (44 million Americans have no health insurance)
• Money for a health club or to join a course devoted to adding physical activity to their daily lifestyle
• Time to join a health club or take a course
• Enthusiasm for adding physical activity to daily living via a structured pay-for program that instructs, monitors, measures, and sets goals

The Small Step Program To Well Being

We have devised a novel approach to one such unstructured program, which we call the Small Step Program To Well Being (Fig. 8–4). The activities shown here are simply examples, rather than absolute recommendations. Indeed, *any* activity can be substituted for the indicated ones, as long as enough activity is accumulated to arrive at the "first big step," which is the minimum amount of physical activity required to start obtaining significant health benefits. Those who are already at the first big step are encouraged to start adding more activity to their daily routines to reach the "second big step," which is the Institute of Medicine's newly recommended goal to accrue additional weight-independent health benefits of physical activity. (These recommendations are elaborated in greater detail later in this chapter.)

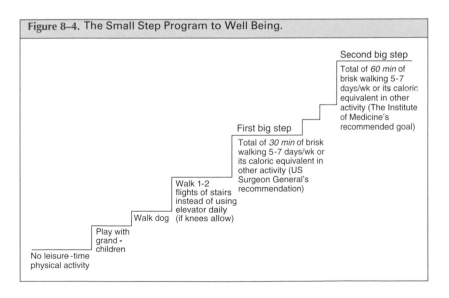

Figure 8–4. The Small Step Program to Well Being.

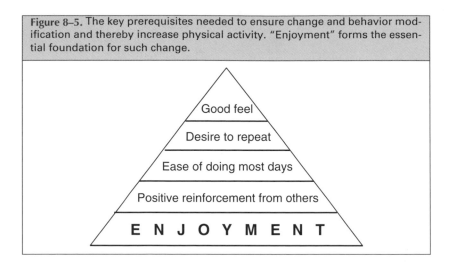

Figure 8-5. The key prerequisites needed to ensure change and behavior modification and thereby increase physical activity. "Enjoyment" forms the essential foundation for such change.

Good feel

Desire to repeat

Ease of doing most days

Positive reinforcement from others

E   N   J   O   Y   M   E   N   T

Such an approach has yet to be proven by a randomized clinical trial. However, given the overwhelming public health benefits to be gained by completely sedentary individuals becoming active, healthcare professionals may wish to employ unproven approaches rather than risk taking a chance with patients' health while awaiting trial results. We believe that anything and everything must be done to transform sedentary patients into physically active ones. There is so much to be gained, and everything to be lost.

Older adults and those less inclined to undertake physical activity (as some persons may be genetically programmed to be inactive) often require structured approaches. These individuals need a lot of prodding, encouragement, and support to increase their level of physical activity. The absolutely necessary incentive is a genuine sense of enjoyment (Fig. 8–5). Innovative programs are still needed.

How To Prescribe Physical Activity

Give prescriptions in a concise and specific manner in terms of the modality, frequency, intensity, and duration (see sample plans below). It is a common misconception that everyone must perform strength, endurance, and flexibility exercises. Remember that to gain health benefits, there is no need for any one specific type of activity. Any type of activity will do (especially for those who are 100% sedentary), as long as 30 minutes of activity (which does not have to be done continuously) is accumulated on most days of the week.

The same physical activity prescriptions cannot be given to every individual. Just as the physician does not treat everyone with hypertension with the exact same medication or dose, and takes into consideration the myriad of factors underlying the individual's condition, one cannot prescribe the same type, intensity, or dose of exercise to all patients. Many factors should be considered before prescribing physical activity. (See Chapter 9 for details on specific counseling issues.)

Case 1: *Many older adults are sedentary, and therefore the first goal is to reduce sedentariness.* Mr. JD is a 75-year-old man with moderately controlled hypertension, type 2 diabetes mellitus, and a BMI of 30. He comes to his internist's office for routine follow-up care. On being asked if he would undertake exercise, he replies: "My knees hurt too much, and besides, I have neither the time nor money to go to a gym". However, Mr. JD does express interest in learning other ways to stay active. During a discussion of his hobbies, he notes that he loves to watch movies and to go to the mall. See Figure 8–6.

Figure 8–6. A physical activity prescription for Mr. JD (Case 1). *Mr. JD could also have been prescribed water aerobics, if he had access to a facility offering such classes (e.g., local YMCA). **Provide instruction and counseling regarding the proper method of performing leg extensions. This also can be accomplished by referring the patient to a physical therapist.

Physician, M.D.
Physical Activity Clinic
USA

Phone: <u>123-555-0000</u>   LIC.# <u>123456</u>

NAME:__Mr. J.D_____   AGE: 75_
ADDRESS:_____ DATE_8/02_

℞

- Decrease the number of hours watching television. Replace by going to movies in mall. While at mall, walk length of mall.
- Park further away in parking lots at stores or malls; take brief walks 2-5 mins during the day as tolerated.*
- Unweighted leg extensions while in front of TV** (to strengthen quadriceps and decrease knee pain)
- Return to clinic in 4 weeks

REFILL___Times

☐ Label

Signature:_____

Case 2: *For those individuals who are already physically active, the goal is to increase the volume of aerobic or resistance activities, and to include a combination of activities to promote variety, which in turn encourages long-term adherence.* Ms. AR is a 60-year-old woman with breast cancer (underwent left mastectomy and chemoradiation, with no disease recurrence in 8 years) and hypothyroidism. She was very active in her teens and twenties, and still likes to hike with her husband. She has otherwise been in good health and has had no other medical problems. Her concern during this office visit with her family physician is to seek advice on "keeping her bones healthy and from going weak." See Figure 8–7.

Here are some tips you can share with your patients to help them add physical activity to their daily routines:

Figure 8–7. A physical activity prescription for Ms. AR (Case 2). *Provide instruction and counseling regarding the proper method for performing resistance exercises and the expected goals. **Fixed weights (weight machines) can also be used as an alternative to ankle weights for lower extremity strengthening exercises, if Ms. AR can afford and access a fitness center or gym. This can also be accomplished by referring the patient to a fitness trainer.

Physician, M.D.
Physical Activity Clinic
USA

Phone: 123-555-0000   LIC.# 123456

NAME:__Ms. AR_____   AGE: 60_
ADDRESS:_____ DATE_8/02_

℞

- Warm up with slow walk and stretch
- A single set of 8-12 repetitions using 8-10 different exercise sets, performed 2-3 times per week. Each repetition should be performed slowly through a full range of motion while avoiding holding one's breath*
- Concentrate on lower extremity resistance exercises (e.g knee extensions using ankle weights)**
- Cool down with slow walk and stretch
- Return to clinic in 6 weeks

REFILL___Times

☐ Label

Signature:_____

- Start low, and go slow.
- Be creative in modifying your lifestyle.
- Decrease time spent watching television.
- Park farther away from your destination.
- Take stairs instead of elevators.
- Take brief, brisk walks several times a day.
- Set easily attainable, short-term goals.
- Increase time spent performing moderate-intensity activity by no more than 5% per week, to an eventual goal of 30 min/day of moderate-intensity activity most days of the week.

Risk Stratification and Screening

Before initiating an activity program, previously completely sedentary individuals must undergo a complete history and physical examination directed at identifying cardiac risk factors, exertional signs/symptoms, and physical limitations. ACSM[7] recommends exercise stress testing for all sedentary or minimally active older adults (men > 45 yr and women > 55 yr) who plan to begin exercising at a vigorous intensity (i.e., > 60% VO_2 max). Here are some other conditions warranting an exercise stress test:
- Known CAD or cardiac symptoms
- Two or more CAD risk factors (hypertension, smoking, hypercholesterolemia, obesity, sedentary lifestyle, family history of early coronary heart disease)
- Diabetes
- Known signs/symptoms of pulmonary or metabolic disease.

There are some contraindications to vigorous physical activity (Table 8–3). However, even patients with these conditions can safely undertake low levels of physical activity once appropriate treatments for the underlying conditions have been initiated. For instance, early exercise-based cardiac rehabilitation has become the mainstay of post-myocardial infarction care. Furthermore, the mere presence of coronary heart disease, type 2 diabetes mellitus, stroke, osteoporosis, depression, dementia, chronic obstructive pulmonary disease, chronic renal insufficiency, peripheral vascular disease, hypertension, or arthritis, is *not*—in and of itself—a contraindication for prescribing regular and routine physical activity. Indeed, it is important for these individuals to engage in physical activity to the greatest extent possible as an *intervention* for their condition. Of course, patients should be counseled to stop physical activity and seek medical advice if they experience major warning signs or symptoms (e.g., chest pain, palpitations, lightheadedness, severe diaphoresis).

Exercise testing is now being used as a measure of a person's fitness level (generally expressed as METs), and consequently as a predictor of

Table 8–3. Some Contraindications To Engaging in Vigorous Physical Activity*	
Absolute Contraindications	**Relative Contraindications**
Recent ECG change or myocardial infraction	Cardiomyopathy
Unstable angina, abdominal aortic aneurysm	Valvular heart disease (e.g., aortic stenosis)
Third-degree heart block, malignant ventricular tachycardia	Complex ventricular ectopy
Acute congestive heart failure, end-stage congestive heart failure	Temporary avoidance is required during treatment of hernias, cataracts, joint injuries, etc.
Uncontrolled hypertension	
Uncontrolled metabolic disease	
Known cerebral aneurysm	
Critical aortic stenosis	
Severe behavioral agitation in response to exercise secondary to dementia, alcohol abuse, neurological or psychiatric issues	

*Aerobic and resistance
Adapted from Pollock ML, Franklin BA, Balady GJ, et al: AHA Science Advisory. Resistance exercise in individuals with and without cardiovascular disease: Benefits, rationale, safety, and prescription. Circulation 101: 828–33, 2000.

mortality. Abnormal exercise test results means increased mortality, with relative risk of death doubling as exercise capacity decreases from > 8 METs to < 5 METs.

Prescribing Physical Activity is a Prime Obligation

Epidemiological reports suggest a possible dose-response relationship between the *intensity* of physical activity and the health benefits accrued from that activity. Results of these studies indicate that going from no regular physical activity to moderate-intensity physical activity (e.g., brisk walking at 4.0–4.5 mph 30 min/day, 5–7 days/wk) has the greatest public health benefit. Dose-response relationships also exist between *increased* physical activity and reduced risk for most chronic diseases—again, the greatest increase in public health benefit is seen when going from sedentary to moderate-intensity activity (Fig. 8–8). Remember that gradually graded increments of activity should be prescribed, especially for those who have been completely sedentary.

Summary

The ability of healthcare professionals to prescribe physical activity and achieve results depends upon their:
  • Understanding of the physiology and scientific basis for long-term adherence to regular physical activity

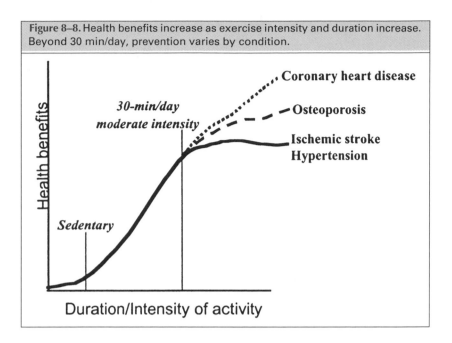

Figure 8–8. Health benefits increase as exercise intensity and duration increase. Beyond 30 min/day, prevention varies by condition.

- Knowledge of the demographics and health status of our present population, and of the ingrained societal influences on exercise behavior
- Access to evidence-based guidelines in concert with training and behavioral programs geared to age-specific barriers and motivational factors.

The precise mechanisms whereby physical activity influences many chronic diseases and modifies risk factors are an area of intense investigation. Despite the obvious need for more research, it is unequivocally clear from numerous epidemiological studies that *patients who are sedentary have significantly greater risks for chronic diseases* than those who engage in regular moderate-intensity physical activity. Therefore, need for future research is *not* a valid excuse for disregarding patients' physical activity levels. (See Chapter 17, Bed Rest/Spinal Cord Injury, for information on the secondary health risks incurred by the inability to undertake physical activity voluntarily.)

As healthcare professionals, we are the primary advocates for our patients' well being. Hence, we also should be positive role models and more proactive in our communities (and at the state level) to promote environmental and policy changes that would facilitate increased physical activity and beneficial health behavior change.

Physical Activity Prescription for Specific Age Groups and Situations*

This statement by Blair and Wei applies to all age groups and situations:

"Inactivity and low fitness are important predictors of health and function in older women and men. The findings generally show a strong dose-response gradient across activity or fitness groups, which include those over 80 years of age. Low activity or fitness appear to be as strong as, or even stronger than, other risk factors such as overweight or obesity, family history, smoking, hypertension, or elevated cholesterol as predictors of morbidity, mortality, and functional status. Based on these findings, practitioners should give increased attention to inactivity and low fitness in medical care and health promotion programs. Many practitioners would never think of not obtaining weight, smoking status, and data on other risk factors from older individuals in their programs, but many of these same individuals would never ask detailed questions about physical activity habits, and few would actually measure fitness. Researchers should extend observational studies on these issues to other populations and intensify efforts to develop and evaluate improved methods of physical activity interventions."[9]

For Completely Sedentary Individuals

Completely sedentary individuals should undertake any type of unstructured activity that can be done within the framework of daily living and routines. One such example of unstructured activity is the Small Steps Program (see Fig. 8–4).

For Already Active Individuals

Patients who are already physically active for ≥ 30 min/day can be advised about the importance of maintaining a minimum threshold (30 min/day) of physical activity for health. The goal should be 100% compliance. The rationale for emphasizing a minimum threshold is simply that health benefit is only obtained at ≥ 30 min/day.

---

* Disclaimer: One of the major objectives of a physical activity prescription is to maximize health benefits (and, therefore, compliance) while minimizing the adverse effects of injury. Toward this end, only general guidelines are available, and they continue to evolve as new studies emerge. The following recommendations are in accordance with the state-of-the-art research that is currently ongoing, but they cannot be comprehensive. Our hope is that they will generate more new ideas and better ways to tackle the crucially important problem of physical inactivity.

Patients who accomplish and maintain the minimum level of physical activity for months should be encouraged to undertake additional daily physical activity. A prescription can be written for this increase. Of note, the Institute of Medicine (IOM) has just concluded that 30 min/day of regular physical activity is insufficient to *maintain body weight* in adults in the recommended BMI range (18.5–25 kg/m^2) and to *fully achieve all health benefits* independent of body weight. The IOM states that *60 min/day* of moderate-intensity physical activity (e.g., walking/jogging at 4–5 mph), is required to prevent weight gain and to accrue additional weight-independent health benefits of physical activity. (Further details on the latest IOM recommendations can be accessed online at http://books.nap.edu/books/0309085373/html/697.html#pagetop).

The IOM has commented that while 60 min/day is more than the 1996 U.S. Surgeon General's Report advises (30 min/day), the IOM recommendation is similar to Canada's *Physical Activity Guide.* The Canadian recommendations for daily physical activity are such that increasing intensities of physical activity are associated with lesser daily durations (Table 8–4).

Some might argue that the IOM's recommendation of 60 min/day of moderate-intensity activity is simply not feasible in light of people's busy lives in the 21st century. Others may point out that that it is difficult to get most sedentary patients to do even a minimum of 30 min/day. Common excuses for not being physically active include lack of time and dislike of any exercise. This is the advantage of the Small Steps Program (see Fig. 8–4), in which the patient "starts low and goes slow" to gradually (over weeks and months) build-up enough momentum to reach the first step of 30 min/day of moderate-intensity activity—or, for those who are already physically active, the second step of 60 min/day.

For those already performing 30 minutes of walking per day, the recommended prescription is:

- Increase the intensity of activity (as long as the higher intensity is tolerated without injuries), *or*

Table 8–4. Canada's Physical Activity Guide: Recommendations for Daily Exercise

Exercise Intensity	Daily Duration of the Exercise	Example
Light	60 minutes	Walking < 3 mph, easy gardening
Moderate	30–60 minutes	Walking > 3 mph, biking, swimming, water aerobics, leaf raking
Vigorous	20–30 minutes	Land aerobics, jogging, hockey, fast swimming, fast dancing, basketball

- Increase the duration (for those who dislike higher intensity) at low intensity.

Alternatively, the patient could add more small steps. For example, he or she could climb stairs more often (take stairs instead of elevators), or take the daily walk in a hilly area. Walking up an elevation can add intensity to a brisk walk of the same duration.

Children/Adolescents

Evidence suggests that prescribing *decreased sedentary time* is as effective or more effective than a prescription for more physical activity. In one study, decreasing sedentary behavior in obese children 8–12 years old caused more weight loss and a greater decrease in percentage of body fat than in those undergoing an exercise intervention.[10] Further, children in the sedentary group increased their liking for high-intensity activity and reported lower caloric intake than did children in the exercise group.

As with adults, children can increase their physical activity by modifying their daily routines. Suggestions made by an expert panel of obesity experts included[11,12]:

- Walking to school instead of riding in motor vehicles*
- Playing with a friend in the afternoon instead of talking on the telephone
- Engaging in unstructured outdoor play, such as going to the park with friends (such activities often are spontaneously vigorous)

In addition, children/adolescents can:

- Swim, dance, and perform martial arts (good for children who dislike team sports)
- Play basketball, walk around the block, and bike with parents or siblings

Adults

The American Heart Association (AHA) has put forth specific guidelines. AHA recommendations for adult **physical activity** include[13]:

- Goal: At least 30 minutes of moderate-intensity physical activity on most, and preferably all, days of the week. (If a patient has suspected cardiovascular, respiratory, metabolic, orthopedic, or neurological disorders, or is middle-aged or older and sedentary, he or she should consult a physician before starting a vigorous exercise program.)

---

* Clinicians should help families address safety issues. Some solutions have hidden benefits, such as when the parent walks the child to school several times a week: the child is safe; the parent benefits from the activity; and the parent and child enjoy some time together.

- Moderate-intensity activities (40–60% of maximum capacity) are equivalent to a brisk walk (15–20 minutes per mile).
- Vigorous-intensity activities (more than 60% of maximum capacity) for 20–40 minutes on 3–5 days per week offer added benefits.
- Resistance training with 8–10 different exercises, 1–2 sets per exercise, and 8–12 repetitions at moderate intensity on 2 or more days per week.
- Include flexibility training and an increase in daily lifestyle activities to round out the regimen.

AHA recommendations for **weight management** include[13]:

- Goal: achieve and maintain desirable weight (BMI 18.5–24.9 kg/m²). When a person's BMI is ≥ 25 kg/m², the waist measurement goal should be ≤ 40 inches for men and ≤ 35 inches for women, since numbers greater than these are a strong predictor for increased risk to develop the metabolic syndrome.
- Manage weight by restricting calories in diet (in consultation with a registered dietician or a nutrition specialist) and increasing caloric expenditure (physical activity) as appropriate.
- For overweight or obese persons, reduce body weight by 10% in the first year of therapy.
- Frailty or advanced age is, in and of itself, *not* a contraindication to physical activity, though specific modifications may be required to accommodate individual situations (e.g., disabilities).

The Elderly

Body composition in the elderly is altered according to the type of physical activity performed (Table 8–5). A combination of aerobic ac-

Table 8–5. Age-Related Change in Body Composition Counteracted By Physical Activity		
Body Composition	**Age-Related Change**	**Physical Activity**
Fat	Increased overall fat mass to age 65, then decreased Increased visceral and truncal mass to age 65, then decreased	Aerobic and resistance activity for those who remain overweight
Muscle	Decreased overall mass Decreased power/strength Preferential loss of type 2 fibers	Resistance activity
Bone	Decreased bone mass and density Increased fragility	Weight-bearing aerobic activity and resistance activity
From Fiatarone Singh MA: Exercise comes of age: Rationale and recommendations for a geriatric exercise prescription. J Gerontol Med Sci 57A:M262-M282, 2002; with permission.		

tivity and resistance training is best; balance or stretching by itself is not beneficial as a sole interventional modality. Consider that an elderly individual may have very low maximal aerobic capacity, and thus walking may be a taxing aerobic activity. This is fine, and should not dissuade you or the patient. If the patient doesn't undertake walking, maximal aerobic capacity will further decrease and ultimately lead to an *inability* to walk, etc. (a vicious cycle).

The safety and efficacy of resistance and balance exercises may lead the physician to encourage substituting them for flexibility exercises. However, increased flexibility supplements all other activities, thereby improving disability. Strength and balance should be addressed before aerobic activity is undertaken, because the elderly experience decreased neuromuscular function, which could be hazardous.

A few simple tests can be done to assess the elderly patient's preparedness for physical activity (previously unpublished observations of MB Brown, Ph.D.):

- Stand on one leg (*balance*)
- Get up out of a chair (one without armrests) five times (*leg strength*)
- Walk 25 feet in less than 7 seconds (*flexibility, balance, vision, strength*)

If the individual is unable to perform any of these tests, then the physical activity prescription would be for continued exercises that improve strength and balance (Table 8–6). Reassess these parameters after a period of time by repeating the above tests. If the individual *is* able to perform the above tests, then aerobic activities can be started and gradually integrated as a routine feature of the physical activity regimen.

The benefits of increased physical activity in older patients are numerous (Table 8–7). Studies in 80- to 100-year-old elderly individuals who exercise have found no reports of serious cardiovascular incidents, myocardial infarctions, sudden death, or exacerbations of type 2 diabetes or hypertension.[15] Even in the oldest old, despite multiple comorbidities and preexisting functional impairment and disability, it is safe to prescribe exercise. Physical activity in these circumstances offers benefits not achievable by a solely pharmacological approach, and many standard medications are associated with adverse effects—especially in the elderly. Also, many older patients can't afford multiple medications, so the substitution of physical activity for a medication of equal benefit may allow the patient to afford food.

Increased intensity of aerobic or resistance activity is as effective as anti-depressant medications for major depression.[16,17] Low-intensity aerobic activity increases quality of life and decreases pain/disability, but without cardiovascular (CV) benefits (moderate intensity is required to obtain CV benefits).[17] Low-intensity lower extremity resistance activity plus balance training results in a dramatic reduction in fall rates.[14]

Table 8–6. Prescribing Physical Activity Goals and Dosage in the Elderly

Type of Physical Activity	Dosage Goal			Safety Considerations
	Frequency	Volume/Duration	Intensity	
Resistance	2–3 days/week	1–3 sets of 8–12 reps; 8–10 major muscle groups	Low-moderate 10 sec/rep, with 1 min rest between sets	• Start low, go slow • No ballistic movements • No valsalva maneuver • Increase weights slowly and progressively, as tolerated
Aerobic	4–7 days/week	30–60 min/ session (doesn't have to be continuous)	Moderate intensity; 40–60% of max exercise capacity (VO$_2$ max), or of max heart rate	• Low-impact activity • Weight-bearing if possible • Increase activity slowly and progressively as tolerated
Flexibility	1–7 days/week	1 sustained 20–40 sec stretch of at least 8–12 major muscle groups	Progressive neuromuscular facilitation techniques*	• Static rather than ballistic movements
Balance	1–7 days/week	1–2 sets of 4–10 exercises of dynamic postures**	Progressive difficulty as tolerated***	• Safe environment needed for close monitoring of dynamic postures • Dynamic rather than static activity • Gradual increase in difficulty as competency assessed and demonstrated

*Neuromuscular facilitation technique involves stretching as far as possible, then relaxing the involved muscles, then attempting to stretch further, and finally holding the maximally stretched position for at least 20 sec.
**Dynamic postures include T'ai Chi movements, standing yoga or ballet movements, tandem walking, standing on one leg, stepping over objects, standing on heels and toes, and walking on compliant surfaces such as a foam mattress.
***Intensity is increased by decreasing other sensory input, such as closing eyes while standing or by perturbing the center of mass, such as holding a heavy object to one side while maintaining balance.
From Fiatarone Singh MA: Exercise comes of age: Rationale and recommendations for a geriatric exercise prescription. J Gerontol Med Sci 57A:M262-M282, 2002; with permission.

Table 8–7. Generalized Recommendations for Physical Activity and Disease Prevention/Treatment

Diseases	Recommended Physical Activity Modality To Affect:				Comments
	Decreased Body Weight/Fat	Increased Muscle Mass & Strength	Decreased Blood Pressure	Decreased LDL-C/TG, Increased HDL-C	
Arthritis	Aerobic	Resistance			Low impact activity
Congestive heart failure	Aerobic	Resistance	Aerobic*	Aerobic Resistance*	Resistance training may be more tolerable if dyspnea severely limits activity. Cardiac cachexia is targeted by resistance training.
Coronary artery disease	Aerobic	Resistance	Aerobic	Aerobic Resistance*	Enhanced metabolic profile from combined physical activity modalities Resistance training may be more tolerable if ischemic threshold is very low.
Depression	Aerobic	Resistance*			Decreases anxiety, improves sleep, increasea self-esteem and self-efficacy Moderate-to high-intensity activity more efficacious than low-intensity exercise in major depression Decreases need for medications with adverse effects (a-blockers, sedatives, etc.)

(continued)

	Recommended Physical Activity Modality To Affect:				
Diseases	Decreased Body Weight/Fat	Increased Muscle Mass & Strength	Decreased Blood Pressure	Decreased LDL-C/TG, Increased HDL-C	Comments
Frailty	Aerobic	Resistance Balance training*			Decreases depression, improves nutritional intake
Osteoporosis	Aerobic	Resistance Balance training			Aerobic exercise should be weight bearing. High-impact activity is best, if tolerated. Resistance training effects are local to muscles contracted.
Pulmonary vascular disease	Aerobic		Aerobic	Aerobic Resistance*	Vascular effect is systemic; thus, upper limb ergometry may be substituted for leg exercise if needed. Resistance activity has less robust effect on claudication. Each session to extend time to claudication
Stroke	Aerobic		Aerobic	Aerobic Resistance*	Combination of modalities most efficacious for overall effect

Table 8–7. Generalized Recommendations for Physical Activity and Disease Prevention/Treatment (Continued)

(continued)

Table 8–7. Generalized Recommendations for Physical Activity and Disease Prevention/Treatment (Continued)

Diseases	Recommended Physical Activity Modality To Affect:				Comments
	Decreased Body Weight/Fat	Increased Muscle Mass & Strength	Decreased Blood Pressure	Decreased LDL-C/TG, Increased HDL-C	
Type 2 diabetes mellitus	Aerobic	Resistance	Aerobic	Aerobic Resistance*	Sufficient aerobic activity expenditure needed to expend at least 1000 kcal/wk. Resistance training maintains lean tissue (muscle and bone) better than aerobic training alone during weight loss.
Urinary stress incontinence		Resistance Balance training			Kegel exercises provide effective resistive activity to strengthen pelvic floor musculature and mobility.
Venous stasis disease		Resistance			Lower-extremity strength training induces muscle contractions and pumps return of fluid via the lymphatics.

*Indicates that the data at present are mainly obtained from observational or experimental studies of the effect of the specific exercise modality on the *risk factors* for the disease or syndrome
From Fiatarone Singh MA: Exercise comes of age: Rationale and recommendations for a geriatric exercise prescription. J Gerontol Med Sci 57A:M262-M282, 2002; with permission.

Adult Obesity—Prescription for *Prevention* of Further Weight Gain in the Obese

Climbing stairs for 1 min/day burns 10 kcal/day. Doing this every day for 365 days, an average weight adult would burn 3650 kcal/year, which translates to 1 pound of fat per year. This formula is only applic-

Table 8–8.	Exercise Distance and Duration Required To Prevent Gaining a Pound of Fat in a Year		
Age	**7-yrs (20 kg)**	**15-yrs (50 kg)**	**Adult (70 kg)**
Amount of activity/day (walking @ 2.5 mph pace)	3000 ft (13.6 min)	1200 ft (5.5 min)	1200 ft (5.5 min)
Amount of calories used	3,600	3,600	3,600

able to *prevention* of weight gain, not for loss of weight. As the body defends against weight loss (see Chapter 7, "Caloric Balance and Expenditure").

To maximally burn calories, the determining quantity is the total distance traversed. Even more calories are burned when the distance traversed is vertical instead of horizontal; i.e., climbing a flight of stairs burns about five times more calories than walking on a flat surface in a given time. One pound of fat contains ~3600 kcal. Therefore, to *prevent* a gain of ~1 lb of fat per year (Table 8–8), the average adult would only have to burn 10 kcal/day for 365 days (~3600 kcal).

Pregnancy and Postpartum

The upper limit of safe physical activity during pregnancy has yet to be determined. One reason is that physical activity limits vary so markedly among pregnant women depending on their health status, physical activity history, and stage of gestation. In general, the current data suggest that moderate levels of regular physical activity during a normal pregnancy pose minimal risk to a woman and her fetus—if the woman is in good health, the pregnancy is monitored, and the physical activity program is modified as necessary. Any physical activity prescription given during pregnancy must be based on common sense, flexibility, individualization, and compromise, while taking into consideration all contraindications (Table 8–9).

Physical Activity Prescription During Pregnancy[21]

Healthy pregnant women can begin or maintain moderate intensity physical activity with potentially minimal negative effects. Activity guidelines must be flexible and individualized, and regular monitoring of the woman and her fetus is required.

Three don'ts to share with your patients:
- Don't get exhausted. Take plenty of rest.
- Don't overheat. Avoid humid and hot temperatures.
- Don't dehydrate. Drink plenty of water.

When starting a physical activity program in a **previously inactive**

| Table 8–9.   Contraindications and Warning Signs In Pregnancy | | |
Absolute Contraindications	Relative Contraindications (require closer medical supervision during exercise)	Warning Signs To Stop Exercise
Ruptured membranes (risk of prolapsed cord)	Anemia (moderate to severe)	Muscle weakness
Premature labor	Overweight (BMI > 25)	Shortness of breath
Undiagnosed vaginal bleeding	Uncontrolled, brittle diabetes	Decreased fetal movements
Suspected fetal distress	Hypertension	Dizziness
Intrauterine growth retardation	Heavy smoker	Amnionitic fluid leakage
Severe maternal heart disease (significant valvular or ischemic heart disease)	History of preterm labor, intrauterine growth retardation, or preeclampsia	Headache (may be early sign of preeclampsia or pregnancy-induced hypertension)
Multiple pregnancies	Significant pulmonary disease	Generalized swelling
Acute infection	Twin pregnancies after 24 weeks or term fundal height measurement reached	Pain of hips, back, or pubic symphysis
Incomplete cervix	Breech presentation	Chest pain
Pregnancy-induced hypertension, preeclampsia	Extremely malnourished or underweight	Calf pain or swelling (need to rule out thrombophlebitis)
	Mild valvular heart disease or significant cardiac arrhythmias	
	Previously sedentary lifestyle	

From Kulpa P: Exercise during pregnancy and postpartum. In Agostini R (ed): Medical and Orthopedic Issues of Active and Athletic Women. Philadelphia, Hanley & Belfus, Inc., 1994, p 192; with permission.

woman, wait until the second trimester to allow closure of the neural tube. Prescribe non-weight-bearing activities such as walking, low-impact aerobics, and water sports. For women who are **already fit,** physical activity can be continued at the pre-pregnancy activity level during the first and second trimesters, but it should not exceed 20–40 min/day and should not be at an intense level. After the 29th week, decrease exercise intensity, duration, and frequency slightly, and exercise after meals to avoid hypoglycemia.

Even fit women should avoid scuba diving, hiking at high altitudes, activities that involve high-risk positions and/or extreme jerking motions, and situations where loss of balance would endanger the mother and fetus. All women should avoid prolonged physical activity in a supine position after the fourth month of pregnancy, when the weight of a pregnant uterus impedes adequate venous return. In general, conservative approaches are best, and common sense must prevail.

The **intensity** of physical activity should be low-to-moderate. Since heart rate is naturally elevated during pregnancy, it cannot be used alone as a reliable monitoring tool for intensity. Rate of perceived exertion is probably a better tool because it is the least affected by gestational adaptations. Also, the "talk test" can be used as a good measure to monitor intensity during pregnancy. The **duration** of physical activity depends on the pre-pregnant maternal state of fitness, the stage of gestation, exercise modality used, intensity, environmental conditions, and the maternal response to physical activity. A reasonable exercise period at moderate intensity is 20–40 minutes; this includes warm-up and cool-down time. A regular routine (3–5 times per week is ideal) with shorter durations (20 minutes) is preferred to sporadic episodes of longer durations.

Monitoring Physical Activity During Pregnancy[21]

Pregnant women should continually monitor how they feel while exercising, and should cease exercise immediately if any symptoms of excessive fatigue, pain, bleeding, gushing vaginal fluid, dizziness, shortness of breath, palpations, faintness, tachycardia, back pain, pubic pain, difficulty walking, decreased fetal movement, or persistent contractions occur or have occurred in the pregnancy. Regular medical monitoring by the physician is essential, as the effect of physical activity on the pregnancy can change throughout gestation. Monitoring the exercise program includes assessing for: sufficient weight gain, increasing symphysis fundal heights according to gestation, and fetal wellness by ultrasound.

Physical Activity During the Postpartum Period[21]

As long as exercising mothers ensure that they have increased their caloric intake sufficiently to meet the increased energy demands of both lactation and exercise (lactation alone requires an extra 500 kcal input of energy daily), no adverse effects on milk quantity, quality, or infant weight gain have been reported, even with high-intensity physical activity. No data definitively shows the ideal time to begin physical activity postpartum. Some suggest as soon as the woman feels her body is ready, and others suggest at least 2–6 weeks of recovery first (the first 6 weeks postpartum is a period of great flux for the female body in terms of hormonal changes, sleep deprivation, breastfeeding, stress, and adjustment). During this period, walking is noted to be the best form of physical activity, but any form of activity is recommended as long as excessive fatigue is avoided. In some studies, women required up to 1 year to regain pre-pregnant fitness levels. Other practical considerations include adequate breast support with a proper exercise bra and avoiding bras with underwire construction, which can compress the milk ducts and lead to plugging.

Benefits reported in breastfeeding women undertaking physical activity include increased energy, decreased fatigue and stress, and decreased incidence of postpartum depression.[22] Interestingly, engaging in an aerobic exercise program of walking, jogging, or cycling 4–6 times/week for 45 min at 60–70% of maximum heart rate resulted in no difference in resting metabolic rate, weight loss, change in proportion of body fat, volume or composition of breast milk, and infant weight gain, compared to those women who were completely sedentary.[23,24] Though the exercising women had greater energy expenditures, they also had increased energy intake. Thus, exercise alone without restricting caloric intake does not increase weight loss and speed up the involutional changes induced by pregnancy. However, the exercising women did have a significant improvement in cardiovascular fitness, compared to their sedentary counterparts. These studies highlight the notion that the postpartum period is *not* the time for rapid weight loss, dehydration, or caloric restriction (especially when exercising and breastfeeding), since a weight loss greater than 1 pound per week results in a loss of lactation.[23]

Physical Disability/Spinal Cord Injuries

Electrically induced walking is not the first priority of individuals with spinal-cord injury, but absence of bowel and bladder control, sexual function, hand function, and breathing are higher priorities.[25] However, once these priorities are met, physical activity and muscle conditioning become important to counter the many inactivity-induced chronic disorders. Currently, a computer-controlled, transcutaneous, reciprocal-pattern electrical activation of leg muscles (hip and knee extensors and knee flexors) can be used for strength-training and cardiovascular conditioning.

The benefits of physical activity include improvements in muscle mass as well as in bladder and bowel function. In addition, reductions in venous thrombosis, skin breakdown, osteoporosis, pathological bone fractures, and spasms result from electrically induced contractions of skeletal muscles.[25] (Additional information on exercise for disabled patients is presented in Chapter 17, "Bed Rest/Spinal Cord Injury." For further consideration of individuals with long-term spinal cord injury, please see ref. 26.)

Suggested Reading

1. Bouxsein ML, Marcus R. Overview of exercise and bone mass. Rheum Dis Clin North Am 20: 787–802, 1994.
2. Kesaniemi YK, Danforth E Jr, Jensen MD, et al. Dose-response issues concerning

physical activity and health: An evidence-based symposium. Med Sci Sports Exerc 33(6 Suppl):S351–358, 2001.

3. Shephard RJ. Absolute versus relative intensity of physical activity in a dose-response context. Med Sci Sports Exerc 33(6 Suppl):S400–418, discussion S419–420, 2001.

4. Thompson PD, Crouse SF, Goodpaster B, et al. The acute versus the chronic response to exercise. Med Sci Sports Exerc 33(6 Suppl):S438–445; discussion S452–453, 2001.

5. American College of Sports Medicine Position Stand. Exercise and physical activity for older adults. Med Sci Sports Exerc 30:992–1008, 1998.

6. Dunn AL, Marcus, BH, Kampert JB, et al. Comparison of lifestyle and structured interventions to increase physical activity and cardiorespiratory fitness: A randomized trial. JAMA 281(4):327–334, 1999.

7. Franklin BA, Whaley MH, Howley ET (eds). ACSM's Guidelines for Exercise Testing and Prescription, 6th ed. Baltimore, Lippincott Williams & Wilkins, 2000.

8. Pollock ML, Franklin BA, Balady GJ, et al. AHA Science Advisory. Resistance exercise in individuals with and without cardiovascular disease: Benefits, rationale, safety, and prescription. Circulation 101:828–33, 2000.

9. Blair SN, Wei M. Sedentary habits, health, and function in older women and men. Am J Health Promot 15:1–8, 2000.

10. Epstein LH, Valoski AM, Vara LS, et al. Effects of decreasing sedentary behavior and increasing activity on weight change in obese children. Health Psychol 14:109–115, 1995.

11. Story MT, et al. Management of child and adolescent obesity: Attitudes, barriers, skills, and training needs among health care professionals. Pediatrics 110(1):210–214, 2002.

12. Jonides L, Buschbacher V, Barlow SE. Management of child and adolescent obesity: Psychological, emotional, and behavioral assessment. Pediatrics 110(1):215–220, 2002.

13. Pearson TA, Blair SN, Daniels SR, et al. AHA Guidelines for Primary Prevention of Cardiovascular Disease and Stroke: 2002 Update: Consensus Panel Guide to Comprehensive Risk Reduction for Adult Patients Without Coronary or Other Atherosclerotic Vascular Diseases. American Heart Association Science Advisory and Coordinating Committee. Circulation 106:388–391, 2002.

14. Fiatarone Singh MA. Exercise comes of age: Rationale and recommendations for a geriatric exercise prescription. J Gerontol Med Sci 57A:M262-M282, 2002.

15. Fiatarone Singh MA, O' Neill EF, Ryan ND, et al. Exercise training and nutritional supplmentation for physical frailty in very elderly people. New Engl J Med 330:1769–1775, 1994.

16. Singh NA, Clements KM, Fiatarone Singh MA. A randomized controlled trial of progressive resistance training in depressed elders. J Gerontol Med Sci 52A:M27–35, 1997.

17. Blumenthal J, Babyak M, Moore K, et al. Effects of exercise training on older patients with major depression. Arch Intern Med. 159:2349–2356, 1999.

18. Wolfe LA, Hall P, Webb KA, et al. Prescription of aerobic exercise during pregnancy. Sports Med 8(5):273, 1989.

19. Paisley JE, Mellion MB. Exercise during pregnancy. Am Fam Physician 38(5):143–150, 1988.

20. American College of Obstetricians and Gynecologists. Exercise during pregnancy and the postnatal period. Washington DC, ACOG, 1985.

21. Stevenson L. Exercise in pregnancy. Can Fam Physician 43:107–111, 1997.

22. Heinz-Schelkun P. Exercise and breast-feeding mothers. Phys Sportsmed 19(4):109–116, 1991.

23. Dewey KG, Lovelady CA, Nommsen-Rivers MS, et al. A randomized study of the effects of aerobic exercise by lactating women on breast milk volume and composition. New Engl J Med 330(7):449–453, 1994.
24. Lovelady CA, Nommsen-Rivers LA, McCrory MA, Dewey KG. Effects of exercise on plasma lipids and metabolism of lactating women. Med Sci Sports Exer 27(1):22–28, 1995.
25. McDonald JW, Sadowsky C. Spinal-cord injury. Lancet 359:417–425, 2002.
26. Kirshblum SC, Groah SL, McKinley WO, et al. Spinal cord injury medicine. 1. Etiology, classification, and acute medical management. Arch Phys Med Rehabil 83(3 Suppl 1):S50–57, S90–98, 2002.

Counseling Patients About Undertaking Physical Activity

chapter 9

This chapter discusses some of the unique challenges encountered in physical activity counseling and provides a framework from which effective counseling strategies may be undertaken. Recent evidence in the literature positively shows that multicomponent interventions combining provider advice with behavioral counseling are significantly helpful in initiating healthy levels of physical activity in previously sedentary patients. A team approach that includes referrals to other allied health specialists (e.g., dieticians, exercise physiologists, psychologists) best facilitates and reinforces long-term maintenance of and adherence to a program of physical activity.

Barriers To Undertaking Physical Activity

General Concepts

Before considering strategies to enhance and promote physical activity, it is important to understand why it is difficult to undertake physical activity in the first place. Several characteristics of present-day society discourage physical activity, including:

1. **Replacement of physical work with machines.** Competitiveness and the desire to make profits have lead to this change, both in the workplace and on farms. Profits improve because of better worker productivity.

2. **Preferential concern about acute health illnesses.** People often are more concerned about missing an appointment the next day because of an unexpected acute illness, such as the flu, than missing years of life at some future indeterminate date because of a chronic disease that is "incubating" in them today. For example, a flu epidemic (a communicable disease, with a fairly rapid and acute onset) causes greater public and medical concern than the epidemics of chronic health conditions (which are indolent, non-communicable diseases, but which nevertheless kill more people per year, and cost significantly more to manage). This sentiment

may contribute to the unwillingness of many to undertake physical activity for general preventive health.

3. **A lack of time to counsel patients** on the positive health benefits of physical activity. Physicians are extremely busy, and they may not wish to devote precious time due to the belief that there is insufficient data on reduction of chronic diseases by physical activity. Additionally, patient disinterest and poor readiness for undertaking exercise means that counseling would not be a brief matter.

4. **A lack of conviction** by patients that physical activity is really necessary for health and a lack of will to substitute physical activity for a labor-saving device that can save time.

There has been a drastic shift in the way we now spend our discretionary time (e.g., TV, computers, internet, video games, movies) vs. 100 years ago (e.g., walking from home to other venues for entertainment, active games). The tasks that used to be done manually (for example, filing papers) can now be done simply by clicking a mouse in front of a computer (Table 9–1). As we move toward an era in which everything can be done in a mechanized fashion, including grocery shopping (or-

Table 9–1. The Elimination of Physical Activity From Our Daily Lives in the 21st Century	
1900 A.D.	**2002 A.D.**
Walking	No sidewalks, electric scooter, motorized walkways, automobile
Riding bike to school	Unsafe streets
Stairs	Elevators, escalators
Sweeping with broom	Vacuuming
Plowing field	Tractor with air conditioning and radio
Picking crops	Mechanized harvesters
Filing papers	Computers
Carrying messages	E-mail, telephone, fax
Washing dishes	Dishwasher
Painting a house with brush	Spray paint
Sawing a tree limb	Power saw
Washing clothes	Washing machine
Hanging clothes out to dry	Dryer
Shoveling snow	Snow blower
Sharpening pencil	Electric pencil sharpener
Walking to library	Internet
Opening cans	Electric can opener

dering food via the internet), there are fewer opportunities for normal, healthy people to remain healthy.

The technological progress humankind has achieved in the last half of the 20th century is phenomenal. It has led us to great productivity and prosperity in practically every field. We are able to accomplish tasks related to food and shelter in minimal time, compared to what was possible three to four generations ago. However, many of these tasks are completed in a sedentary manner. It is important that we use some of our saved time to engage in more physical tasks, such as walking, to preserve our health.

The bottom line is that sedentary occupations will never be eliminated from our society. They are here to stay. Since work environments are unlikely to change, most of the change will need to occur during our discretionary time. Thus, participation in regular physical activity must be inculcated into the framework of our daily routines.

Patient-Centered Barriers

Currently ~70% of U.S. adults either do not undertake physical activity or are under-active, and nearly half of America's youth (aged 12 to 21 years) are not vigorously active on a regular basis. If physical activity is such a potent primary preventive medicine, why isn't it more popular? One possibility is that the word "exercise" elicits a negative response in many people. Exercise may suggest intense activity that is associated with pain, specialized equipment, or membership in a health club. Also, some individuals may have negative feelings about exercise due to experiences as children and teenagers if their lack of athletic abilities evoked ridicule from peers.

While health clubs and personal trainers serve a purpose for some individuals, not everyone can afford health clubs or enjoys them. Those who are not club members can still increase their physical activity, but they must recognize barriers in their daily lives that hinder them from doing so (Table 9–2). These barriers include:

- Improper and unsafe transportation routes—
  No sidewalks
  No bike lanes
  Bike lanes too close to traffic
  Bike surfaces with holes to cause accidents
  Crime or fear of crime while walking or cycling
- Unsafe storage for bikes—
  Lack of bike racks or improper placement of bike racks
  Stolen bikes
  Lack of crime prevention by police
- Lack of adequate exercise facilities at worksites—
  Exercise facility only open during working hours

Table 9–2.	Suggestions For Eliminating Many of the Common Barriers To Becoming More Physically Active
Barrier	**Suggested Approach**
Self-efficacy	Begin slowly to build confidence, progress gradually in small steps; provide frequent positive reinforcement and encouragement. Start with low duration and build based upon enjoyment.
Attitude	Promote positive personal benefits of exercise; identify activities that are enjoyed and emphasize internal rewards
Discomfort	Vary intensity and type (cross-training and variety) of exercise. Start slowly. Avoid reaching an intensity that encourages negative reinforcement. Progress slowly toward those durations and intensities to cause some physiological and hormonal responses. Focus on how patient feels after a few minutes of moderate physical activity—the "euphoria" that often accompanies a good exercise session is reinforcing.
Fear of injury	Balance and strength training if patient is very frail; use appropriate clothing, equipment and supervision; start slowly
Habit	Incorporate into daily routine; repeat encouragement; promote active lifestyle within the context of daily living
Subjective norms	Educate patient and family regarding health benefits of exercise; discuss cultural beliefs and biases
Fixed income	Undertake walking and other simple exercises; use household mechanical tasks for physical activity; promote active lifestyle within the context of daily living, i.e., "functional physical activity" (see below)
Environmental factors (e.g. weather, closed facilities)	Walk in the mall (many malls open early to accommodate walkers in the morning); use senior centers, YMCA
Illness/fatigue	Use a range of exercises that patients can match to their ability to perform physical activity without discomfort; stretching exercises—start slow and progress gradually
Time limitation	Build into daily routines; promote active lifestyle within framework of daily living; educate regarding many positive benefits of physical activity; take time for enhancing personal well being and health. Time recommended (minimum) is only 30 min, 5+ days per week (i.e., 2.5 to 3 hours per week).

Closed on weekends, holidays, and vacations

No showering facility in workplace (needed if arriving via running or cycling)

- Weather—rain, snow, ice, cold, heat, tornado warnings cancel outside physical activity
- Crime or fear of crime—unsafe locations for physical activity

- Exercise-related injury—cancels physical activity (person may be unaware that alternate forms of activity can be taken up and substituted).
- Cost to join an exercise facility—
    Don't have the money or don't wish to spend the money
    Perception that physical activity can only be done in a health club
- Perception that physical activity is not necessary—
    Elderly men and women commonly assert that regular physical activity is not necessary at their age; they frequently have unrealistic expectations regarding the health benefits of their daily activities, and they seriously exaggerate the risks of vigorous exercise.
    Lack of understanding regarding the effects of physical inactivity on long-term health
    Heavy individuals tend to overestimate their physical activity by almost 40%
- Pain and cultural beliefs—
    Notion of avoiding anything that hurts (physical activity at moderate levels and performed properly does not hurt)
    Some women may think it "unfeminine" or "unladylike" to exercise
- Poor self esteem—
    Embarrassed by poor athletic skills
    Misperception that one must train as hard as a role model elite athlete to get a health benefit

Functional physical activity is that which is part of everyday errands and tasks. Ironically, actual time inventories find that people have 24–25 hours of discretionary time per week! Thus the time barrier is false, especially when one considers the numerous opportunities to engage in functional physical activity (see first column, Table 9–1). We suggest that instead of approaching physical activity as a time-consuming ordeal, physicians should explain to their sedentary patients that walking or bicycling 10–15 minutes twice a day instead of driving a short distance, parking on the far side of the mall instead of driving around for the closest space, using stairs, doing yard work, playing with children or grandchildren, and restricting time watching TV will all be beneficial.

We think the term "well being" should replace "fitness" to describe why increasing physical activity is important for keeping healthy. The average layperson relates fitness to athletics and not to well being or health. If the aim is to enhance patient health, then the term that will elicit a greater adherence to prescriptions of physical activity should be used.

Physician-Centered Barriers

The Writing Group for the Activity Counseling Trial (ACT) noted that: "The role of physicians and other health care practitioners in advising sedentary patients to become physically active is recognized by national organizations, but there are numerous barriers to counseling these patients."[2] A recent report[3] found that the three leading barriers to physicians prescribing and counseling increased physical activity were:

1. Inadequate time for dedicated patient education and counseling to encourage physical activity

2. Lack of necessary skills and tools for providing such counseling

3. Lack of reimbursement from health-insurance and managed-care plans for physical activity–related preventive health maintenance and treatment programs.

These barriers are significant. Despite the obvious evidence supporting the numerous benefits of physical activity in preventing chronic health conditions, it is ironic that only 18–48% of patients (depending on the study) are advised to increase their level of physical activity. Physicians seem to predominantly counsel physical activity as a form of *secondary* prevention, as evidenced by higher counseling rates in patients who are already obese, who are older than 30 years, or who have comorbid conditions, and lower counseling rates in groups at high risk for obesity, weight gain, and sedentary lifestyle.[4] In addition, there is a failure to counsel younger, disease-free, and sedentary adults as well as those from lower socioeconomic groups. These are important **missed opportunities** for primary prevention, which could lead to adverse public health outcomes.

It may be argued that additional randomized controlled clinical trials are needed to evaluate the precise effectiveness of physician-mediated physical activity counseling and interventions (especially in groups at risk for not having discussions about physical activity with their physicians). However, given that the problems directly associated with a sedentary lifestyle have now reached epidemic proportions in the U.S., even modest benefits from relatively benign interventions, such as counseling to increase physical activity in the sedentary, would have a markedly substantial public health impact.[4]

Features That Contribute To Difficulty Counseling Physical Activity

Healthcare professional's perspective[3]:
1. Lack of reimbursement
2. Limited time for counseling—

- Prescription of physical activity takes more time and effort to perform than prescribing a pill.
- Exercise prescriptions must be more detailed, in contrast to brief drug prescriptions. Patients must be told more than just "go and exercise more."
3. Limited training to counsel appropriate physical activity—
   - It is a misconception that a decline in physical activity is a natural part of the aging process. Physical inactivity speeds the functional decline of organ systems with aging, whereas activity delays this decline in most organs (see Chapter 16, "Aging").
   - Lack of knowledge regarding how to write physical activity prescriptions.

Patient's perspective[5]:
1. Difficult to find time for physical activity in busy schedule—
   - Physical activity requires more time than taking a pill.
   - The patient is solely responsible. Others can prepare low-fat meals and administer pills, but they cannot perform physical activity for the patient.
2. Patient's lack of understanding about the health benefits of physical activity—
   - The public accepts heavily advertised pharmaceutical modalities, but does not similarly accept that physical activity has great therapeutic benefits.
   - Physical activity is thought of as a purely recreational or competitive activity, rather than as a potent therapeutic or prophylactic regimen.
   - Many people associate exercise with hard labor, for which they don't see an immediate, tangible benefit. They decide that they don't want to use their leisure time "working." Some believe that "exercise for exercise's sake is frivolous."
   - Those who participated in competitive events may have difficulty exercising without a trophy at stake.
3. Delayed gratification—
   - Pills and potions often have immediate effects, whereas the results of physical activity are only noticeable over time and are not as obvious (e.g., rapid resolution of pain with an analgesic or of fever with an antipyretic vs. a disease prevented years from now).
   - The deadly consequences of not engaging in physical activity are not readily apparent: for example, diabetes and heart disease, which are directly linked to physical inactivity, span many decades before their destructive effects become manifest. In contrast, noncompliance with pharmaceutical regimens often has swift and unpleasant consequences.

Guidelines For Physical Activity Counseling

Healthcare professionals can successfully inspire sedentary individuals to become physically active by increasing their awareness of the many tools and counseling strategies that have proved helpful. After a review of the many intervention studies,[10–12] we conclude that the more intensive and sustained the counseling strategy, the greater its effectiveness.

Here are the **U.S. Preventive Services Task Force (USPSTF) Guidelines** for physical activity counseling[6]:

1. Ask questions about the patient's physical activity level during the history-taking on routine healthcare visits.

2. Identify inactive patients who do not appear to meet the minimum level of physical activity associated with gains in cardiorespiratory fitness: intensity of 50–100% maximal oxygen uptake, duration of 15–45 min, and frequency of 2–4 times/week. It has been repeatedly found that moderate-intensity exercise (analogous to brisk walking) on most (preferably all) days of the week provides significant health benefit to sedentary populations, and the U.S. Surgeon General now prescribes this activity.

3. Attempt to interest sedentary patients in adopting a program of regular physical activity by discussing the role of physical activity in disease prevention and by addressing the patient's individual risk of conditions associated with inactivity. Also determine the patient's perception of his or her health status.

4. Guide the patient in choosing an appropriate type of physical activity that would be efficacious for health, such as:

- Activity that is predominately weight-bearing, if not contraindicated
- Results in energy expenditure
- Contributes to cardiovascular fitness
- Has a low potential for adverse effects
- Effective for adherence
- Activity with moderate intensity
- Low perceived exertion
- Low cost
- Convenient
- Close to home
- Flexible time and location
- Lack of need for specialized facilities
- Opportunity for social interaction
- The potential for incorporation into routine daily activities.

Walking is an optimal physical activity for sedentary patients. Seventy-six percent of the individuals in the National Weight Control Registry[23] used walking as their preferred form of physical activity and walked 21–28 miles per week. These 3000+ subjects lost 66 lbs and kept it off for 6 years.

5. Guide the patient in choosing an appropriate level of participation. The initial level should be only a small increment above baseline status. Gradual progression should occur over a period of weeks to months, with a goal of reaching the minimum level outlined above (see no. 2). Familiarize the patient with measuring pulse rate during exercise, and set appropriate goals for intensity, duration, and frequency based on estimating the maximal O_2 uptake according to heart rate. The maximal heart rate can be crudely estimated by subtracting one's age in years from 220. Some patients may have trouble with the concept of the pulse rate, as they can't consistently find their pulse, count it wrong, etc. Thus, an alternative approach is to use an inexpensive heart rate monitor. Encourage patients at each visit to set at least one specific goal for intensity, duration, and frequency that can be built upon in the future. An exercise diary may be useful for this purpose.

6. Monitor compliance with physical activity, and provide positive reinforcement during future healthcare visits.

7. Discourage big increases in physical activity, which increase risk of injury and adverse effects and sometimes lead to noncompliance. Advise patients to consult their physician if they encounter persistent injury or adverse effects (see Chapter 8 for the American College of Sports Medicine Guidelines on exercise stress testing with physician supervision).

8. Encourage the social support of significant others.

9. Identify barriers to optimal adherence, and discuss strategies for overcoming them.

10. Encourage physical activity adherence, particularly after major lifestyle transitions, such as graduation for high school or college, marriage, job change, residence change, or recovery from illness or injury ("relapse training" is crucial, and additional encouragement prevents individuals from completely stopping regular physical activity).

11. An exercise electrocardiogram is not necessary for asymptomatic, generally healthy persons planning to increase their level of physical activity from sedentary to moderate-intensity walking. However, the Physical Activity Readiness Questionnaire can be useful in identifying persons needing special medical attention.

The **Physical Activity Readiness Questionnaire**[6]:
- Has a doctor ever said you had heart trouble?
- Do you frequently have pains in your heart and chest?
- Do you often feel faint or have spells of severe dizziness?
- Has a doctor ever said your blood pressure is too high?

- Has a doctor ever told you that you have a bone or joint problem such as arthritis that has been aggravated by exercise, or might be made worse by exercise?
- Is there a good physical reason not mentioned above why you should not follow an activity program even if you wanted to?
- Are you over age 65 and not accustomed to vigorous exercise?

Clinical Evidence For Efficacy of Physical Activity Counseling

The current clinical evidence is mixed. Even though the USPSTF provided counseling guidelines, the very same organization also concluded in their most recent report[7] that behavioral counseling to encourage physical activity in primary care settings has mixed effectiveness, especially in terms of sustained increases in regular physical activity in adult patients. However, the USPSTF concluded that the effectiveness of primary care clinician counseling would be enhanced by: (1) combining provider advice with intensive, multi-component interventions and behavioral counseling strategies (such as written exercise prescriptions, individually tailored physical activity regimens and goal setting, and mailed or telephone follow-up assistance provided by specially trained staff), and (2) referring patients to other allied heathcare specialists and community-based physical activity and fitness programs.

It is important to note that these USPSTF conclusions were based only on a review of the literature evidence for the effectiveness of physical activity counseling in *primary care settings.* Most of the reviewed studies focused on brief, minimal, low-intensity primary care interventions, such as a 3- to 5-minute counseling session at the end of a routine clinical visit amidst addressing other complex medical issues of the patient. In fact, there is ample evidence in *non-primary-care settings* that show the effectiveness of physical activity counseling in increasing and sustaining routine physical activity.

Various Counseling Programs Effectively Promote Daily Physical Activity

While the USPSTF addressed the effectiveness of *individual clinician counseling* in primary care settings to increase physical activity, the Task Force on Community Preventive Services[8] addressed the effectiveness of *community-based programs* that target groups rather than individual patients. This Task Force found a number of interventions to be effective, including community-wide campaigns, changes in school-based physical education programs, improved access to places for physical activity, and individually based behavior change programs. (More details on these interventions are presented in Chapter 11, "Promotion of Routine Daily Physical Activity.")

Several organizations (U.S. Dept Heath and Human Services [Healthy People 2010], U.S. Centers for Disease Control and Prevention, American Academy of Family Physicians, American Academy of Pediatrics, American Heart Association, and American College of Obstetricians and Gynecologists) unequivocally recommend that healthcare providers counsel patients about physical activity.[7] However, the USPSTF cautions that these recommendations are based only on the perceived health benefits of physical activity, and not on the effectiveness of individual provider counseling to promote changes in physical activity. The USPSTF acknowledged that the effectiveness of individual clinician counseling would be enhanced by multi-component interventional programs applying intensive counseling strategies in conjunction with other allied healthcare expertise (e.g., fitness trainers). Indeed, programs that establish individual goals, teach skills for incorporating physical activity into daily routines, provide problem-solving techniques, and reinforce motivation have been found to be the most successful in initiating and maintaining regular physical activity.

The Activity Counseling Trial

The Activity Counseling Trial (ACT)[2] is an excellent example of a multi-component intervention that includes written and tailored physical activity prescriptions, as well as close follow-up. This randomized, controlled clinical trial assessed three treatment groups: standard care, staff assistance, and staff counseling. The latter was the most intensive treatment regimen of the three (Table 9–3).

Using this wide array of methods, several of the interventional objectives and behavioral changes were accomplished (Table 9–4). Note the complexity and the highly intensive multi-modal treatment regimens involved in behavior modification. The results obtained from the ACT underscore the fact that an intensive counseling regimen given by both physicians and other staff members (e.g., dieticians, RNs, exercise physiologists, psychologists) using a multi-modal approach is needed over an extended period of time, and that the brief, 3- to 5-minute intervention or follow-up, as is commonly done in routine primary care clinical encounters, is likely going to be ineffective in increasing the level of physical activity in most sedentary patients.

The ACT is significant because it is truly one of the first randomized, controlled trials to clearly show a remarkable benefit and efficacy of primary care counseling to increase the level of physical activity above that of a sedentary baseline. Twenty-two contacts with 50-year-old healthy patients for physical activity counseling (totaling 3 hours of counseling

Table 9–3.   Interventions in the Three ACT Treatment Groups

| Intervention Components | Experimental Treatments | | |
	Standard Care (A)	Staff Assistance (B)	Staff Counseling (C)
Initial encounter			
Physician advice	Yes	Yes	Yes
Written materials	Limited	Yes	Yes
Mail-back cards	No	Yes	Yes
Behavioral video	No	Yes	Yes
Personal counseling	No	Yes	Yes
Schedule behavioral change classes	No	No	Yes
Schedule additional in-person sessions	No	No	Yes
Mailing components			
Monthly newsletters	No	Yes	Yes
Mail-back cards	No	Yes	Yes
Incentives for returning mail-back cards		Yes	Yes
Feedback sheets	No	Yes	Yes
Telephone components			
Patient-initiated calls	Limited to exercise type and amount	Yes	Yes
Calls every 6 months	No	Yes (only to reestablish contact)	Yes
Counselor-initiated calls	No	One	Monthly or more
Regular telephone counseling	No	No	Yes
Subsequent clinic visits			
Physician advice	No	Yes	Yes
Personal counseling at physician visits	Limited as above	Yes	Yes
Ongoing classes	No	No	Yes
Individual counseling sessions	No	No	Yes
Other components			
Home visits	No	No	Possible

Adapted from Writing Group for the Activity Counseling Trail Research Group: Effects of physical actvitiy counseling in primary care. The Activity Counseling Trial: A randomized controlled trial. JAMA 286: 677–687, 2001.

per patient by visits, calls, and newsletters) in primary care practices over 2 years resulted in a dramatic increase in the percentage of people undertaking ≥ 30 min/day of moderate-intensity physical activity 5–7 days/week, from 1–2% at baseline to 26% after 24 months.

Table 9–4. How Behavioral Change Was Effected in the Activity Counseling Trial		
Theory-Based Mediators of Behavioral Change	**Intervention Objective**	**ACT Experimental Treatments***
Personal variables		
Performance	Achieve a series of realistic short-term goals	Newsletters and mail-back cards (B,C). Phone counseling/ classes (C).
Barriers	Identify internal and external barriers that make it difficult to be active	Video (B,C); Newsletters & tip sheets (B); Phone counseling/ classes (C).
Outcomes expectancy	Develop realistic expectations	Exercise booklet & physician counseling (A,B,C); Video (B); Newsletters, & tip sheets (B); Phone counseling/classes (C).
Incentives		
Perceived benefits	Identify personal benefits of being active; make them salient	Exercise booklet & physician counseling (A,B,C); Video, newsletters & tip sheets (B,C); Phone counseling/ classes (C).
Enjoyment	Select enjoyable activities and do them in comfortable settings	Exercise booklet & physician counseling (A,B); Video, newsletters & tip sheets (B,C); Phone counseling/ classes (C).
Rewards for achievements	Identify intrinsic and extrinsic rewards that will motivate change	Physician counseling (A,B); Newsletters & tip sheets (B,C); Phone counseling/classes (C).
Self-regulatory skills		
Problem-solving	Develop plans for overcoming barriers; implement plans	Newsletters & tip sheets (B); Phone counseling/classes (C).
Self-monitoring/ feedback	Regularly record levels of physical activity; receive regular feedback on progress	Step counter & monthly calender; mail-back cards & tip sheet graphs (B,C); Phone counseling/ classes (C).
Self-evaluation	See self as an active person; based on self-monitoring records, set and revise goals to increase activity	Video, newsletters, mail-back cards & tip sheets (B,C); Phone counseling/classes (C).
Self-reinforcement	Provide rewards to self when goals are met; use self praise	Newsletters (B); Phone counseling/classes (C).
Relapse management	Expect occasional slips; make plans for anticipated barriers; re-start activity after slips (opportunities to learn)	Newsletters & tip sheets (B, C); Phone counseling/classes (C).

(continued)

Theory-Based Mediators of Behavioral Change	Intervention Objective	ACT Experimental Treatments*
Table 9–4. How Behavioral Change Was Effected in the Activity Counseling Trial (Continued)		
Social variables		
Modeling of activity	Observe, interact with others who lead active lives	Video & newsletters (B, C); Phone counseling/classes (C).
Support for physical activity	Ask family, friends, coworkers to assist with, or participate in, activities; receive support & assistance from intervention health educators & personal physician	Physician counseling (A, B); Video & newsletters (B, C); Phone counseling/classes (C).
Physical environment variables		
Access to facilities	Become more familiar with local facilities, such as health clubs, walking & biking trails	Resource guide & newsletters with inserts; Phone counseling/classes (C).
Access to resources that promote activity	Stay informed about local activity-related events, clubs, services	Resource guide & newsletters with inserts; Phone counseling/classes (C).
Access to programs	Become more familiar with local programs, such as aerobics classes, swimming lessons, walking groups	Resource guide & newsletters with inserts; Phone counseling/classes (C).
Stages of change		
Readiness to change or increase activities; Relevant information or skills	Examine your motivation; obtain relevant information or skills	Physician counseling (A, B, C); Newsletters, mail-back cards, & tip sheets (B, C); Phone counseling/classes (C).

*A = standard care, B = staff assistance, C = staff counseling
Adapted from Writing Group for the Actvity Counseling Trail Research Group: Effects of physical actvitiy counseling in primary care. The Activity Counseling Trial: A randomized controlled trial. JAMA 286:677–687, 2001.

Summary of the Clinical Evidence

While the USPSTF concludes, based on a review of only the primary care literature, that the efficacy of physical activity counseling by a single provider in the primary care setting (where other medical treatment decisions for the patient are also being made) is mixed, numerous other studies, including the ACT trial, have clearly shown that intensive counseling strategies are highly efficacious. Indeed, even the USPSTF recommendations acknowledge that if any counseling strategy would be promising, it would be that which integrates physician advice with intensive multi-component behavioral interventions that are undertaken in concert with a wide array of other healthcare professionals, and which includes referrals to community-based physical activity and fitness programs, and not a counseling strategy that entails only a 3- to 5-minute, rushed counseling session at the end of a routine clinic visit.

We realize that the employment of such intensive measures will not be easy or practical in all situations. A drastic change in our outlook and perhaps even a reprioritization of healthcare objectives may need to occur. Consider that there is already a paradigm set up for such a process to happen even in a routine, brief clinical encounter in the primary care setting, as evidenced by the frequent use of referral services by the primary care clinician. For example, if a specialized test needs to be done for a patient, or an opinion needs to be obtained for a vital treatment decision, or a diabetic patients needs education on diet and various types of insulin preparations, primary physicians frequently call upon consulting and support staff services, even though the essential care is being orchestrated by the primary care provider. In much the same way, the various aspects of physical activity counseling need to be delegated to a team of specialists and support staff, while coordinated by the clinician. Such delegation may facilitate tailoring the counseling to the specific situation or circumstance of the individual patient, and this can be done over an extended period of time.

In addition, though the USPSTF recommendations note that it is still unclear whether routine follow-up by primary care physicians results in increased physical activity among adult patients, it is our opinion that assessing compliance and adherence, and incorporating the recommendations of the various consultants can only benefit the patient. An idea for overcoming the time constraints associated with routine follow-up in primary care settings is to have specialized "physical activity promotion clinics" or "preventive medicine clinics," where the focus of the visit is purely high-intensity counseling and behavior modification. The session is initiated by the primary provider and then reinforced by the other support staff in the clinic. Such clinics already exist in other medical fields (e.g., preventive cardiology clinics). Of course, these programs require time, money, and personnel allocations, as well as proper use of the various behavioral counseling tools.

We think that the issue of limited resources is a matter of perspective. The U.S. spends almost a *trillion dollars a year* to treat and diagnose diseases. Yet, amazingly, 50% of all deaths in the U.S. are completely preventable![24] Healthcare costs are expected to double by 2011, so cost reduction must be undertaken. It is our contention that allocation of resources to the aforementioned endeavors would not only save the U.S. economy a lot of money in the long run, but also would keep people healthy longer and out of hospitals and nursing homes, as well as improve their quality of life.

Given that sedentary behaviors have contributed directly to the epidemics of chronic diseases in our current society, we really do not have a choice but to advocate for maximal counseling and promotion of increased physical activity and other health behavior change. In our view, not doing so constitutes a direct violation of one of the central tenets of the Hippocratic oath, i.e., do no harm.

In many ways, counseling to increase physical activity is similar to that for smoking cessation, with the usual pitfalls and success rates. The clinical benefit in having people stop smoking directly results in them living longer. The same applies to counseling sedentary people to become more physically active.

One of the common excuses given for minimal physical activity counseling by primary care practitioners (besides time constraints) is inadequate knowledge of the various behavior-modification tools (see Table 9–4). The following text outlines some common behavioral strategies that have proven to be efficacious. A primary care practitioner can use them individually or in conjunction with other support staff. At the very least, goals should include identifying patients who are ready to undergo behavior change/modification, referring them appropriately, and following closely.

Mechanics and Strategies of Behavior Modification

Assess each individual's state of **readiness for change** (Fig. 9–1). The Stages of Change Model is based on the transtheoretical model and social cognitive theory.[9,10] *Without motivation, effort will not be forthcoming.* Patient motivation is the key component for undertaking and adhering to physical activity.

Counseling may be targeted or tailored. **Targeting** means that the focus is on a largely homogenous population group. Individuals in the group are similar enough (in terms of characteristics, motivation, preparation, etc.) to be influenced by the same message.[11] **Tailoring** means that the message is given to one specific person, based on the characteristics unique to that one individual. Time spent on assessment, the level of personalization, and participant effort are all much greater than in targeting.[11]

As elucidated by Napolitano and Marcus,[12] though tailoring and targeting are used in interchangeable ways, they have markedly different features that separate them and form a central core of each counseling

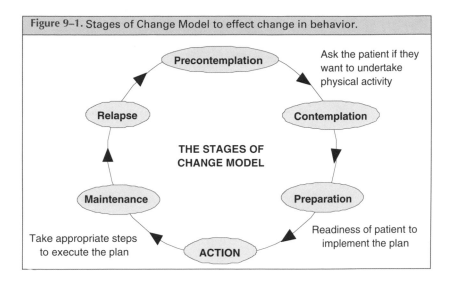

Figure 9–1. Stages of Change Model to effect change in behavior.

Precontemplation

Ask the patient if they want to undertake physical activity

Relapse

Contemplation

THE STAGES OF CHANGE MODEL

Maintenance

Preparation

Take appropriate steps to execute the plan

ACTION

Readiness of patient to implement the plan

strategy. Studies by Marcus et al[10] have shown that physical activity counseling given in a tailored setting (i.e., tailoring the message based on where the individual is in the Stage of Change Model) compared to a standard setting (where the group receives the message via self-help booklets developed by the AHA) results in a significantly greater number (43.6% vs. 18.1%) of people reaching—and exceeding—the CDC/ACSM recommended physical activity criteria. The patients in the study by Marcus et al also increased the duration of their physical activity. Other behavioral studies have proven that feedback and counseling based on individualized approaches (Table 9–5) are more effective than a more generic, "one-size-fits-all" approach.[11]

Algorithms can also be helpful in assessing patient readiness to undertake, or to increase, physical activity (Fig. 9–2) and in determining counseling strategy. The physician should take a "physical activity history."

There is currently no information to address how much individualization and specificity for both targeted and tailored interventions are necessary for maximum levels of behavior change in physical activity. There also is limited information regarding the optimal dose of tailoring, the important variables on which to tailor, and number of contacts needed. More research is necessary.

Follow-Up

Each office visit should be an opportunity for evaluation of progress and assessment of the following, as established initially:

- Patient's exercise goals—examine and adjust periodically according to progress

Table 9–5. Examples of How To Tailor Messages Based On the Stage of Change Model	
Stages of Change	**Counseling Topics & Tips**
Precontemplation	Topics include *defining the problem*; assessing readiness; benefits and barriers of physical activity; assessing self-efficacy and confidence level; raising consciousness about physical activity by giving information related to caloric balance, use of proper shoes, injury prevention, etc. *Examples:* "Our goal is to help you find ways to make physical activity a more regular part of your life." "How ready are you?"
Contemplation	Topics similar to precontemplation, but emphasis is on *developing definite plans to become more active,* rewards, using reminders, and goal setting. *Examples:* "As you pay more attention to the advantages of being physically active, you will find it easier to take steps towards being active on a regular basis." "Congratulations on your efforts!"
Preparation	Topics similar to contemplation, but emphasis is on *trying to identify and overcome barriers. Example:* "Remember that everybody faces unexpected situations that make undertaking physical activity difficult, such as bad weather and family situations, but the key is to keep it going."
Action	Topics similar to the first 3 stages, with increased emphasis on *building confidence in undertaking the proposed activities,* in addition to goal setting and overcoming barriers. *Examples:* "Believing in yourself and making commitments to be active are important ideas that can help you achieve your goals." "Continue with the goals you have set." "Congratulations on your efforts!"
Maintenance	Topics include the same themes as in the first 4 stages, but with the emphasis on *extending confidence levels and staying motivated. Examples:* "You've been learning a lot about the benefits of physical activity and have continued being regularly active. That's great! It's important to notice how far you've come in achieving your goals." "You've also made great progress in keeping things in your environment that motivate you to be active; magazines and posters concerned with physical activity can be great sources of inspiration." "Keep walking shoes by the door." "Keep up the good work!"
Relapse	Topics are the same as in the preceding 5 stages, with the emphasis now on *self-reevaluation, stimulus control, problem solving, and self-reinforcement. Examples:* "Note that everybody faces situations that cause them to slip into inactivity. You can use these situations as learning experiences, and think about what caused the slip; then you can try something new the next time instead of repeat the same mistakes. Learn to avoid the places and things that encourage you to be inactive." "Rewards can be a great source of motivation, and

(continued)

Table 9–5.	Examples of How To Tailor Messages Based On the Stage of Change Model *(Continued)*
Stages of Change	**Counseling Topics & Tips**
	can be accomplished simply by the things you say to yourself when you go for a walk or when you read about exercise." "Think about all of the positive things that physical activity does for you, that initially made you get into it in the first place: your body feels better, you sleep more soundly at night, and you have more energy and vitality during the day. So keep thinking positively!"

Adapted from Napolitano MA, Marcus BH: Targeting and tailoring physical activity information using print and information technologies. Exer Sports Sci Rev 30(3): 122–128, 2002.

- Self-monitoring and modifying thoughts during activity—address any pain or discomfort and monitor for any evidence of injury
- Increase social support

Note that encouragement and positive reinforcement should be given for the slightest signs of improvement. Additionally, even in a

Figure 9–2. Algorithm to assist in discussions with the patient about issues related to physical activity. (Adapted from Christmas C, Andersen RA. Exercise and older patients: guidelines for the clinician. J Am Geriatr Soc 48: 318–324, 2000.)

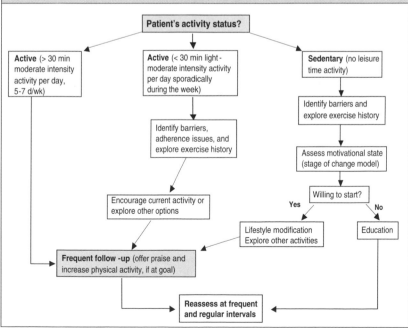

time-constrained primary care setting, follow-up can be used to discuss and incorporate the recommendations (obtained during previous visits) of the various consultants and support staff, thereby engaging the patients in the counseling and behavior modification process. By caring for the patient in this way, he or she receives a potent, positive message that reinforces new behaviors. Endorsement by the primary care provider carries great weight.

Adherence

1. Determine the patient's needs and expectations.
   - Systematic planning is imperative during the formative stages of an intervention to ensure that the participant's needs and expectations are met.
   - Conduct initial and follow-up interviews.
2. Help the patient to develop self-regulatory skills.
   - Goal setting is facilitated by the understanding that physical activity is a behavior directed toward a purposeful end, rather than a threat or source of frustration.
   - Short-term goals must be set as small steps to attain the larger goals.
   - Environmental modifications should be explored in advance, such as alternate locations for exercising during inclement weather and ways to engage in physical activity when traveling.
3. View physical activity as a continuum and an ongoing dynamic process, rather than a static behavior.[5]
   - Goals and expectations must be constantly reviewed and revisited, with new goals and expectations set. Relapse prevention must be part of the planning process, and relapses should be described as expected occurrences that interrupt, rather than terminate, physical activity. Emphasize to patients that "lapses" (missed sessions of physical activity) do not mean "collapse"!
   - Motivation fluctuates over time, with periods of varying commitment and enthusiasm. Frequent reassessment also is helpful in maintaining long-term goals and adhering to physical activity over time.
   - Be cognizant of the fact that people have preferences as to whether they undertake physical activity in a structured setting (fitness center), or unstructured setting (park or neighborhood). Some require social interaction while engaging in exercise, whereas others favor solitude.
4. Use phone contacts; they are invaluable tools for maintaining adherence.
   - Periodic calls provide encouragement, affirmation, social sup-

port, and verbal rewards, as well as the opportunity to discuss problems and frustrations impeding the maintenance of physical activity.

- Programs such as INTERVENT (www.interventusa.com) involve phone contacts on a regular basis with patients (see Chapter 11 for more details).

5. Help the patient to associate positive feelings with exercise.
- The patient can partner with a friend.
- Partners can arrange to report progress to each other.
- The exercising individual should aim to increase self-efficacy; this is the key to success. As he or she continues to exercise, confidence will grow.
- Focus on post-exercise euphoria.
- Pay attention to fitness gains. These are the obvious, even visual benefits of physical activity.

Avoid "One-Size-Fits-All" Counseling

A systematic approach to counseling includes a realistic physical activity prescription, if the plan is to be successful (see Chapter 8, "Physical Activity Prescription"). Additionally, the patient should be educated not only about various general health benefits, but also about the *specific* benefits available to him or her, keeping in mind the patient's goals and level of motivation (i.e., location in the Stages of Change Model). Obtain a history of physical activity. Counsel your patient to:

- Set goals. Accumulate ≥ 30 min of moderate intensity physical activity on most, if not all, days of the week. Determine how you are going to get there, and how you will know you've arrived.
- Overcome inertia. Have realistic expectations; start slow and increase slowly.
- Self-monitor. Post reminders about being physically active. Think of yourself as an active person.
- Self-reward. Such reinforcement can be a powerful source of motivation, and it doesn't always have to be a material item.
- Manage time well. Incorporate activity into your lifestyle, and make it a priority.
- Monitor thoughts during activity. Try to avoid negative thinking.
- Use "slips" as learning experiences.
- Make physical activity interesting and come up with creative ways to make it more fun.
- Increase social support. Find a helper; talk with someone; go for a walk with friends.

Several behavioral studies[10–13] have shown that individually tailored approaches result in the greatest positive behavior changes, compared to generic, "one-size-fits-all" approaches. There is no question that the former are costly in terms of time, money, resources, etc. But given the alternative (i.e. the rapidly rising mortality and economic costs associated with the epidemic of chronic diseases), as well as the plethora of epidemiological studies unequivocally demonstrating the positive benefits of physical activity in preventing disease, such an investment is worthwhile and, indeed, justified and necessary.

Counseling Strategies for Children/Adolescents

Obtaining a Pediatric Physical Activity History

Two different expert panels have suggested specific sets of questions to better assess and counsel appropriate levels of physical activity in children/adolescents.

1. Expert Panel of obesity experts convened by the Maternal and Child Health Bureau, Health Resources and Services Administration, and the Department of Health and Human Services[15]:

What physical activities were done?
- Quantify vigorous activity, such as organized sports and school-based physical education.
- Activities in daily living, such as walking to school or to the bus stop, unorganized outdoor play, yard work, and household chores.

What is the sedentary time activity?
- Television-viewing, reading, computer and video games, etc
- How much time is spent in a sedentary fashion?

What are deterrents to activity?
- Unsafe neighborhoods
- Lack of adult supervision after school
- Lack of equipment/facilities

What alliances might provide supervision/support in increasing physical activity?
- Parents
- Caregivers

2. American Heart Association's Scientific Statement[16]:
- How much time is regularly spent walking, bicycling, and in backyard play? Using stairs, playgrounds, and gymnasiums? Playing interactively and physically with other children?
- What is the number of hours spent per day in sedentary leisure activities?
- How much time is spent participating in age-appropriate organized sports, lessons, clubs, or league games?
- In school or day-care physical education that includes a mini-

mum of 30 minutes of coordinated large-muscle exercise (for children > 2 years of age)?
- Participating in household chores?
- On family outings that involve walking, cycling, swimming, or other recreational activities?
- Is there a positive role model for a physically active lifestyle (e.g., parents, other caretakers, physicians, school personnel)?

The AHA also states that the following should be considered:
- Child's age, sex, race, and level of sexual maturity
- Physical and mental disabilities that may affect exercise participation (i.e., chronic diseases or medical conditions)
- Familial attitudes toward exercise and sport participation; also socioeconomic and environmental factors
- Child's access to convenient places for exercise
- The ability of the family to encourage regular activity.

AHA Guidelines for Pediatric Physical Activity Counseling

These guidelines can help you to formally address the subject of exercise in your practice[16]:
- Advise parents to include planned activities instead of food as part of the family's reward system for positive accomplishments.
- Advise parents to establish time limits for sedentary activities and encourage a daily time for physical activity.
- Emphasize the benefits of regular physical activity: an improved cardiovascular risk factor profile, increased energy expenditure, improved weight control, a general sense of physical well-being, improved interpersonal skills, and an outlet for psychological tension.
- Do not include or exclude a child from activities because of physical or mental limitations. Tailor suggestions for physical activity to the child's physical ability.
- Encourage participation in pick-up games, noncompetitive activities, and organized sports. Emphasize sports that can be enjoyed throughout life, participation in summer camp, and school physical education programs.
- Make suggestions appropriate to the age of the child.
- Incorporate advocacy of physical education into your role as a school health professional, if applicable. Make sure all children are involved.
- Teach parents the importance of being role models for active lifestyles and providing children with opportunities for increased physical activity.
- Be an advocate for physical health in your community.

Strategies for Decreasing Sedentary Behaviors

Decreasing sedentary behavior is a primary prevention against pediatric obesity. There are several approaches:

1. Family-based (parents can participate with their children)
   - Outdoor time together
   - Walking to school
   - Walking on errands
2. School-based
   - Promotion of recesses
   - Physical education that provides equal opportunity for fun activity regardless of athletic ability. De-emphasize fitness and winning. Fitness will naturally follow voluntary playing for fun.
3. Children's sports leagues
4. Other[17]
   - Since obesity is likely a consequence of pervasive influences that operate across many settings, the development of effective preventive interventions likely requires strategies that affect multiple settings simultaneously.
   - Expect the external pressures that encourage eating and sedentary occupations to continue.
   - Decrease caloric intake (take home part of a large restaurant meal to consume as a second, "leftovers" meal for the next day).
   - Increase caloric output (encourage children to play with other children outside, if safe).

Primary prevention involves getting children away from sedentary events and allowing spontaneous play. Toward this end, counsel parents to abide by the guidelines of the American Pediatric Association to limit TV watching to ≤ 2 hours. These guidelines should be posted in every pediatrician's office, and parents should receive these guidelines with mailings. Minimal daily increases in physical activity in children significantly prevents/attenuates gains in body fat when caloric intake is maintained/unchanged.

The Paradox of Child Safety

Paradoxically, children may be in harm's way while playing outside, but their health is also at risk if they spend excessive time in front of the TV. We realize that limiting TV hours may be difficult for some parents because TV can occupy a child and keep him or her "safe" from crime outside. Consider, however, that the child is compromised by physical inactivity. TV limits indoor play, which consequently diminishes the time parents must spend monitoring indoor play or listening to the child. As documented earlier (see Chapter 5), hours of TV watching are directly associated with an increase in obesity.

We suggest that healthcare professionals advise parents to make a "safe" room for child play. This room can be used when the TV-watching time limit of the American Academy of Pediatrics is met. Also, neighboring parents can share supervision by having children alternate play between houses on different days. It is possible that such indoor play will not be active enough, but this is a starting point for children who are completely sedentary.

Counseling Strategies for Adults

Obtaining an Adult Physical Activity History

Ask the following questions[13]:

What is the patient's lifelong pattern of activities and interests?
- A person who has never been physically active is less likely to initiate and maintain a high-intensity program.
- An ex-endurance athlete is likely to be comfortable engaging in and maintaining a regular physical activity program.

What has been the patient's activity level in the past 2–3 months?
- Establish a current baseline.
- Use the baseline to guide initiation of activity and ascertain changes with time.

What are the patient's concerns and perceived barriers regarding physical activity?
- This is by far the most useful part of the history. (Barriers are explored in detail earlier in this chapter.) The most common barrier to undertaking regular physical activity is patients' perception that they don't have time. Yet, according to CDC and ACSM recommendations, only 30 minutes of moderate-intensity physical activity on most, if not all, days of the week is sufficient (remember, continuous, uninterrupted activity is *not* required) to gain many health benefits.
- Note that health benefits from regular physical activity can be accrued even without losing weight. Thus, from a purely health maintenance perspective, it is as important and useful to counsel the obese patient to be more physically active, as to lose weight.

What is the patient's level of interest and motivation for exercise?
- This question establishes a starting point for the physical activity prescription plan.
- Repeated assessments raise the patient's awareness of the problem and convey a strong message that physical activity is important for optimizing healthy living.

What are the patient's social preferences regarding exercise?
- Individuals must be empowered to make active decisions and

be involved in their exercise prescription to ensure greater adherence.

- Also, a social setting (such as undertaking physical activity with a friend or relative) and endorsement of a family member (spouse) affords greater adherence and motivation.

Tailor Counseling To Each Individual

After documenting the above historical features and determining the motivational state of the individual, give a clear and specific exercise recommendation (preferably on a prescription pad, much in the same way a prescription for a medication is given). See Figures 8–6 and 8–7 in the previous chapter.

Adherence and benefits from increased fitness are maximized by customizing the exercise prescription for each individual. Take into account the following elements while writing the physical activity plan:

What would *you* like to have the patient do?

What would *the patient* like to do?

How much time is available for physical activity?

What is the activity history of the individual?

Are social, cultural, and environmental factors a problem?

Are equipment and facilities available?

Be sure to assess comorbidities and other functional limitations that may limit the patient's ability to perform certain types of activity.

Counseling Strategies for the Elderly

Effective physical activity interventions are not always successful in promoting health in the elderly, as this population often does not comply with recommendations and, in general, does not continue increased physical activity in the long-term. In one study, while high participation rates were achieved with short-term physical activity interventions (< 1 year), long-term interventions (> 1 year) showed lower participation rates.[18] Possible explanations for the inverse relationship between the participation rate and length of intervention could be lack of interest, motivation, enjoyment, time, or perceived benefits.[18] The best success rate was achieved in group-based interventions, followed by home-based interventions, with educational-based interventions being the least effective in older adults. Nevertheless, despite relatively poor success rates of physical activity counseling in the elderly, continued efforts are strongly recommended—especially in light of the tremendous public health benefits and public policy implications.

Consider the following when counseling elderly patients:

- Alternatives to traditional group-based interventions, such as

helping older adults to exercise at home, during leisure time, and in competition-oriented activities
- Reoccurrence of sedentary behaviors
- More intense long-term strategies to promote long-term changes in lifestyle, such as: safe community design, community-level resources, workplace promotion efforts, counseling in healthcare delivery systems, and education
- Tailoring interventions to individuals' ideas and preferences
- A variety of physical activity options
- Frequent contacts with the elderly patient.

Recognize that professional assistance and support may be needed for more complex counseling situations. Sometimes, working one-on-one with an older adult who needs to be more physically active but has special needs (e.g., a chronic disease such as type 2 diabetes, hypertension, arthritis) may be warranted. Many elderly patients find that it hurts to move, so they set up a cycle wherein pain yields more inactivity and inactivity yields more pain. Another barrier for the elderly may be financial: a special facility for one-on-one support may be too expensive.

Competent personal health and physical activity consultants and programs like INTERVENT (http://www.interventusa.com) can help overcome these difficulties (see Chapter 11, "Promotion of Routine Physical Activity"). Such programs are also effective models for behavior change[19] and have been useful in increasing physical activity levels in patients with chronic diseases. INTERVENT and similar approaches focus on intensive and sustained counseling strategies delivered by on-site, phone, and internet methods.

Counseling and Goal Monitoring for Specific Types of Physical Activity

1. Aerobic activities
   - "Start low and go slow"
   - Warm up by slow-walking for 5 min and stretch slowly for 5 min, then walk (briskly), bicycle, and/or swim at moderate intensity for a cumulative total of 30 min
   - Cool down by walking slowly and stretching again to improve flexibility and decrease risk of injury
   - *Increase the duration by no more than 5% per week.*
2. Resistance activities
   - "Start low and go slow"
   - Warm up by slow-walking for 5 min and stretch slowly for 5 min
   - *Goal is to lift a weight that is 70–80% of a one-repetition maximum*

(or the most one can lift though a full range of motion once), 8–12 repetitions per set for a total of three sets, with 1–2 min of rest between sets

- Proper breathing during these exercises is vital: Exhale during the lift for 2–4 sec and inhale during the lowering of the weight for 4–6 sec, working though the entire range of motion. This will avoid contraction of the abdominal muscles against a closed glottis (i.e., prevent Valsalva maneuver) during lifting and lowering of the weights, which can lead to decreased venous return to the right side of the heart and consequent hypotension.
- Cool down by walking slowly and stretching again to improve flexibility and decrease risk of injury.
- *Increase resistance when the previous weight sets become easy.*
- Refer patients to health clubs and certified personal trainers.
- Bring weights to the patient's home (especially the elderly).
- Keep a log of the weights lifted, and record body weight once or twice a month. Do not overdo weights.

Counseling By Specific Disease

Two disease examples—obesity and diabetes—are arbitrarily chosen for illustration, mainly because of the preponderance of recommendations in the current literature. Healthcare professionals should assess **overweight/obesity** and recommend weight loss (using the combination of a low-calorie diet and increased physical activity) to overweight and obese patients. Weight maintenance should be recommended to patients with normal weight.[20] In a study by Galuska et al, only about 40% of obese persons having a routine checkup had been counseled by healthcare professionals to lose weight. Persons who are advised to lose weight by their medical caregivers are more likely to attempt to lose weight than those who are not so advised.[21,23] Therefore, physicians, nurses, and others must make it a priority to actively counsel patients regarding weight control and management.

All patients with **type 2 diabetes** should have a complete history and physical examination prior to starting a physical activity regimen. Pay particular attention to evaluation of cardiovascular disease, medications that may affect glycemic control during or after exercise, and diabetic complications including retinopathy, nephropathy, and neuropathy. This is necessary because people with type 2 diabetes often find it difficult to exercise and are at increased risk for injury or exacerbation of underlying diseases or diabetic complications.[22] If a patient has had a recent treadmill test, the results can be used to issue specific physical activity prescriptions, especially for those who like a more structured program. Emphasize to patients with type 2 diabetes that the magnitude of the physical activity's effects on glycemic control, insulin sensitivity, and risk factors for cardiovascular disease must be considered in determining the feasibility and acceptability of a physical activity intervention program; the type and duration of physical activity is less important.[22]

Suggested Reading

1. Nied RJ, Franklin B. Promoting and prescribing exercise for the elderly. Am Fam Phys 65:419–426, 2002.
2. Writing Group for the Actvity Counseling Trail Research Group. Effects of physical activity counseling in primary care: The Activity Counseling Trial. JAMA 286:677–687, 2001.
3. Petrella RJ, Wright D. An office-based instrument for exercise counseling and prescription in primary care: The Step Test Exercise Prescription (STEP). Arch Fam Med 9:339–344, 2000.
4. Wee CC, McCarthy EP, Davis RB, Phillips RS. Physician counseling about exercise. JAMA 282:1583, 1999.
5. Chao D, Foy CG, Farmer D. Exercise adherence among older adults: Challenges and strategies. Controlled Clin Trials 21:212S–217S, 2000.
6. Harris SS, Caspersen CJ, DeFriese GH, Estes EH Jr. Physical activity counseling for healthy adults as a primary preventive intervention in the clinical setting. Report for the U.S. Preventive Services Task Force. JAMA 261:3588–98, 1989.
7. USPSTF writing group. Behavioral counseling in primary care to promote physical activity: Recommendations and rationale. Ann Int Med 137:205–207, 2002.
8. Recommendations to increase physical activity in communities. Am J Prev Med 22(4 suppl):67–72, 2002.
9. Bandura A. Self efficacy: The exercise of control. New York, WH Freeman and Company, 1997.
10. Marcus BH, Bock BC, Pinto BM, et al. Efficacy of an individualized, motivationally tailored physical activity intervention. Ann Behav Med 20:174–180, 1998.
11. Kreuter MW, et al. One size does not fit all: The case for tailoring print materials. Ann Behav Med 21:273–283, 1999.
12. Napolitano MA, Marcus BH. Targeting and tailoring physical activity information using print and information technologies. Exer Sports Sci Rev 30(3):122–128, 2002.
13. Christmas C, Andersen RA. Exercise and older patients: Guidelines for the clinician. J Am Geriatr Soc 48:318–324, 2000.
14. Stevens M, Bult P, de Greef MH, et al. Groningen Active Living Model (GALM): Stimulating physical activity in sedentary older adults. Prev Med 29:267–276, 1999.
15. Barlow SE, Dietz WH. Obesity evaluation and treatment: Expert Committee recommendations. The Maternal and Child Health Bureau, Health Resources and Services Administration and the Department of Health and Human Services. Pedriatics 102:E29, 1998.
16. Williams CL, Hayman LL, Daniels SR, et al. Cardiovascular Health in Childhood: A Statement for Health Professionals From the Committee on Atherosclerosis, Hypertension, and Obesity in the Young (AHOY) of the Council on Cardiovascular Disease in the Young, American Heart Association. Circulation 106:143–160, 2002.
17. Dietz WH, Gortmaker SL Preventing obesity in children and adolescents. Annu Rev Public Health 22:337–353, 2001.

18. van der Bij AK, Laurant MG, Wensing M. Effectiveness of physical activity interventions for older adults: A review. Am J Prev Med 22:120–133, 2002.
19. Franklin B, Bonzheim K, Warren J, et al. Effects of a contemporary, exercise-based rehabilitation and cardiovascular risk-reduction program on coronary patients with abnormal baseline risk factors. Chest 122:338–343, 2002.
20. National Heart, Lung, and Blood Institute. Clinical Guidelines on the Identification, Evaluation, and Treatment of Overweight and Obesity in Adults: The Evidence Report. Washington, DC, U.S. Government Printing Office, 1998.
21. Galuska DA, Will JC, Serdula MK, Ford ES. Are health care professionals advising obese patients to lose weight? JAMA 282: 1576–1578, 1999.
22. Hamdy O, Goodyear LJ, Horton ES. Diet and exercise in type 2 diabetes mellitus. Endocrinol Metab Clin North Am 30:883–907, 2001.
23. Wing RR, Hill JO. Successful weight loss maintenance. Annu Rev Nutr 21:323–341, 2001.
24. Hoffman C, Rice D, Sung HY. Persons with chronic conditions. Their prevalence and costs. JAMA 276:1473–1479, 1996.

Management of Overweight and Obesity

chapter

10

Prevalence of Overweight/Obesity

In the United States, approximately 60% of adults and 25% of youth are overweight/obese. Prevalence has doubled in a 10-year period in children, adolescents, and adults. The Centers for Disease Control calls obesity an epidemic. Obesity is more prevalent in minority populations, especially Afro-American, Hispanic, and Native American. Thirty-five percent of Afro-American and Hispanic children and 20% of Caucasian children are overweight (BMI $>$ 85th percentile for their age). Overweight/obesity and its comorbid conditions affect $>$ 100 million Americans, accounting for more than $100 billion of all direct and indirect medical costs. Yet the prevalence of the disorder continues to increase.

Another disturbing statistic was reported by Kimm et al[11]: levels of physical activity decline so precipitously in adolescent girls in the United States that by the age of 18 years the majority are engaged in virtually *no* habitual physical activities. Factors underlying the physical activity decline in adolescents were found to be BMI (for each 1 unit increase in BMI, physical activity decreased 0.8 MET-time/wk), pregnancy (a major factor in African-Americans), smoking, parents with only a high-school education level, and lack of a mother or father (single parent). Increasing sedentariness in our youth should cause great concern, since childhood/adolescent obesity portends grave consequences in adulthood in terms of developing morbid chronic diseases. We healthcare professionals must take immediate steps to curb obesity and to inculcate physical activity and healthy behaviors during our children's early years.

The increase in obesity over the last 30 years is due to caloric imbalance, i.e., eating more and expending less in physical activity. Although sometimes postulated as a cause, there have been no new gene mutations in the past 30 years in millions of unrelated individuals and ethic groups.

Diseases and Disorders Stemming From Overweight/Obesity

Obesity leads to multiple co-morbidities, which increase the overall risk of dying (Fig. 10–1). Obesity increases deaths from cardiovascular disease (Fig. 10–2) and cancer (Fig. 10–3). In one study, the 10-year risk of developing diabetes increased with increasing BMI in both men and women, with 6% and 5% developing diabetes, respectively (Fig. 10–4).[2,3] The 10-year risk of developing hypertension also increased with increasing BMI in both men and women, with 13% and 14% developing hypertension, respectively (Fig. 10–5).[2,4] The same was true for

Figure 10–1. All-cause mortality from obesity. *Dashed line* = women, *solid line* = men. (Adapted from Calle EE, Thun MJ, Petrelli JM, et al: Body-mass index and mortality in a prospective cohort of U.S. adults. N Engl J Med 341:1097–1105, 1999.)

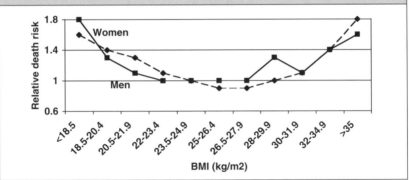

Figure 10–2. Cardiovascular deaths from obesity. *Dashed line* = women, *solid line* = men. (Adapted from Calle EE, Thun MJ, Petrelli JM, et al: Body-mass index and mortality in a prospective cohort of U.S. adults. N Engl J Med 341:1097–1105, 1999.)

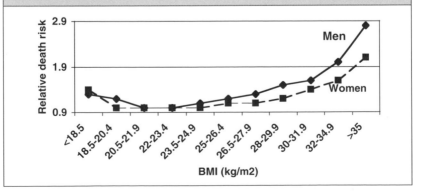

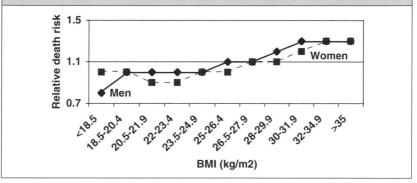

Figure 10–3. Cancer deaths from obesity. *Dashed line* = women, *solid line* = men. (Adapted from Calle EE, Thun MJ, Petrelli JM, et al: Body-mass index and mortality in a prospective cohort of U.S. adults. N Engl J Med 341:1097–1105, 1999.)

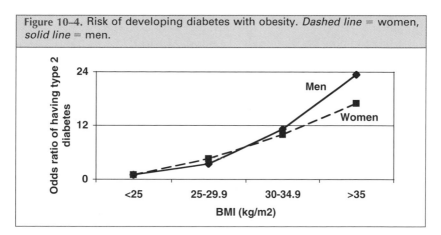

Figure 10–4. Risk of developing diabetes with obesity. *Dashed line* = women, *solid line* = men.

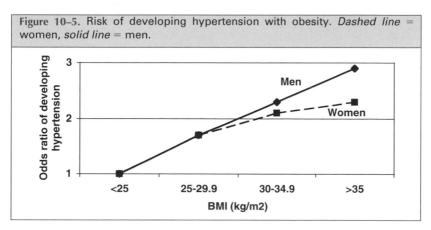

Figure 10–5. Risk of developing hypertension with obesity. *Dashed line* = women, *solid line* = men.

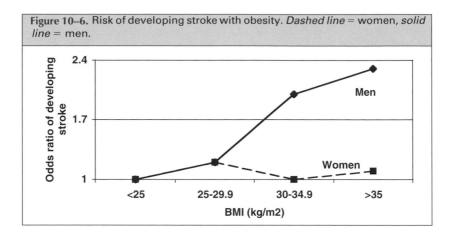

Figure 10–6. Risk of developing stroke with obesity. *Dashed line* = women, *solid line* = men.

stroke, with the risk increasing significantly more in men compared to women (Fig. 10–6).[2,5]

Life-threatening co-morbidities of obesity include:

- Established coronary heart disease (MI, angina)
- Peripheral arterial disease
- Abdominal aortic aneurysm
- Symptomatic carotid artery disease
- Sleep apnea

Diseases associated with obesity that require detection and appropriate management, but that generally do not lead to widespread or life-threatening consequences include:

- Gynecological abnormalities (polycystic ovary syndrome)
- Osteoarthritis
- Gallstones and their complications
- Stress incontinence

Co-morbidities occurring with pediatric obesity are delineated in Chapter 5.

Assessment of Adult Body Weight

Body weight and height: see Figure 10–7.

Body mass index: BMI measures weight in relation to height (Table 10–1). BMI = weight (kg)/height (m^2). The health risk increases at higher levels of overweight and obesity. BMI calculators are available at http://www.nhlbisupport.com/bmi/ and http://www.cdc.gov/nccdphp/dnpa/bmi/calc-bmi.htm.

Waist circumference: The greater the intra-abdominal fat (visceral fat), the higher the risk of cardiovascular disease and type 2 diabetes

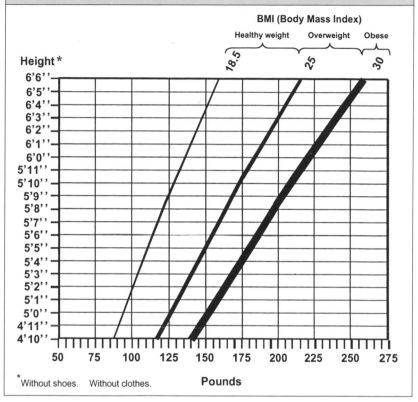

Figure 10–7. Adult weight-for-height chart. Directions for determining your BMI: Find your weight on the bottom of the graph. Go straight up from that point until you come to the line that matches your height. The intersecting point identifies your health status and BMI. (Data adapted from http://www.nhlbi.nih.gov/guidelines/obesity/bmi_tbl.htm.)

mellitus. Multiple metabolic disturbances associated with abdominal obesity include glucose intolerance, hyperinsulinemia, insulin resistance, hypertension, and dyslipoproteinemia, now widely known as the metabolic syndrome. Waist circumference > 40 inches in males and >

Table 10–1. Adult Body Mass Index Chart		
Weight Classification	Obesity Class	BMI (kg/m²)
Underweight		< 18.5
Normal		18.5–24.9
Overweight		25.0–29.9
Obesity	I	30.0–34.9
	II	35.0–39.9
Morbid obesity	III	≥ 40

Table 10–2. Classification of Overweight and Obesity By BMI, Waist Circumference, and Associated Disease Risk*				
			Disease Risk* Relative to Normal Weight and Waist Circumference	
Weight Classification	BMI (kg/m²)	Obesity Class	Men ≤40 inches Women ≤35 inches	Men > 40 inches Women > 35 inches
Underweight	< 18.5		—	—
Normal	18.5–24.9		—	—
Overweight	25.0–29.9		Increases	High
Obese	30.0–34.9	I	High	Very high
	35.0–39.9	II	Very high	Very high
Morbidly obese	≥40	III	Extremely high	Extremely high

* Hypertension , dyslipidemia, type 2 diabetes mellitus, coronary artery disease, stroke, gallbladder disease, osteoarthritis, obstructive sleep apnea
Data from http://www.nhlbi.nih.gov/guidelines.

35 inches in females is considered a high risk for morbidity. Weight loss is recommended to preserve health in such individuals.

For risk stratification of various adult body weight assessments, examine the classifications offered by the National Institutes of Health (Table 10–2).

Assessment of Pediatric Body Weight

Use one of the charts prepared by the Centers for Disease Control (Fig. 10–8 or Fig. 10–9) to determine whether the child/adolescent is obese (body size is in the upper 95th percentile) or overweight (body size is in the 85th–95th percentile). Enter the individual's age on the x-axis and the calculated BMI on the y-axis, and then identify the percentile from the intercepting curved line.

Barriers To Effective Assessment of Obesity

Unfortunately, obesity often is not recognized as a chronic, complex condition that is difficult to treat. As a result, healthcare professionals may be unaware that long-term management strategies are required, and that relapse rates are high. Other barriers to effective assessment of obesity include:
- Insufficient clinic time for counseling
- Insufficient data on the effectiveness of physician-mediated weight loss counseling
- Inadequate training in the medical management of obesity

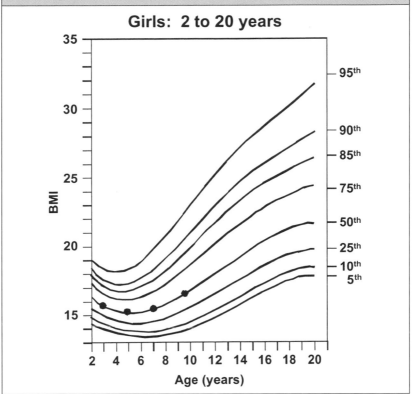

Figure 10–8. Chart showing body mass index-for-age percentiles for girls. For example, the same girl would be in the 50th percentile of her age group at 3, 5, 7, and 9 years of age if her BMIs were 15.7, 15.1, 15.4, and 16.5, respectively (*black dots*). (Data adapted from http://www.cdc.gov/nccdphp/dnpa/bmi/bmi-for-age.htm.)

Girls: 2 to 20 years

- Lack of reimbursement from insurance companies for obesity-related programs.

Counseling For Weight Loss and Management

Obese individuals do not need to achieve optimal body weight for health benefits, since even modest reductions of 5–10% have significant health benefits. The issues are losing weight and maintaining the loss in the overweight/obese and preventing gain in normal-weight individuals. Multidimensional counseling strategies that include all ancillary health-care staff (e.g., registered nurses, registered dietitians, exercise physiologists, behavior therapists) are needed.

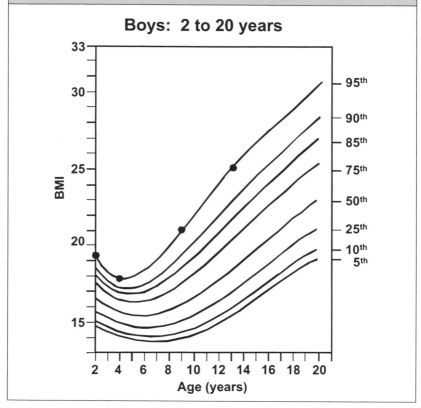

Figure 10–9. Chart showing body mass index-for-age percentiles for boys. For example, the same boy would be in the 95th percentile of body weight for his age with BMIs of 19.3, 17.8, 21.0, and 25.1 at the ages of 2, 4, 9, and 13 years, respectively (*black dots*). (Data adapted from http://www.cdc.gov/nccdphp/dnpa/bmi/bmi-for-age.htm.)

Overweight/Obese

Why Is Counseling Essential?

Counseling remains the central component in any weight management program for obese patients. Obese patients who receive counseling and weight management from physicians are significantly more likely to undertake weight management programs than those who do not.[12] However, the success of weight loss is highly dependent on the patient's self-motivation level. Therefore, key objectives of weight counseling are to (1) assess the patient's motivation to lose weight, and (2) help him or her to achieve a change of motivational state. Considering the high stakes and the tremendous burden of obesity, taking the time for such counseling is worth it.

Unfortunately, counseling for weight loss tends to be sought mainly by those in the higher socioeconomic bracket and those who have achieved higher levels of education. These are the same individuals who are likely to be insured and therefore regularly visiting healthcare professionals; for this reason they are more likely to be offered advice on weight loss and management. Ironically, the greatest incidence of obesity occurs in the *lower* socioeconomic bracket and in individuals at *lower* educational levels!

Goals of Counseling in Overweight/Obese Patients

Goals for loss:
- ~ 10% of baseline weight in 6 mo (or ~1–2 lbs/wk, with a caloric deficit of 500–1000 kcal/day)
- Losing weight faster has not shown to be of more benefit, since the faster weight is lost, the faster it is regained.
- For long-term weight loss, it is best to decrease at the rate of 1–2 lbs/wk.

Goals for maintenance:
- It is easier to lose 5–10% of body weight than to maintain this weight loss after 1 year.
- After 6 months, the priority of counseling should be to *maintain* the new weight. Encourage increased physical activity and/or decreased caloric intake.
- A combination of modalities may be more effective in helping the patient maintain the new weight.

Nutrition counseling:
- The key is to use moderate reductions in caloric intake to achieve a slow but progressive weight loss.
- A low-calorie diet (800–1500 kcal/day) is better than a very-low-calorie diet (250–800 kcal/day). The latter is unsuccessful in achieving long-term weight loss, and also is nutritionally unsound, with increased risk of developing gall stones.
- Select a nutrient composition that will decrease other risk factors such as increased cholesterol and hypertension.
- Low-calorie diets can decrease total body weight by an average of 8% and help decrease abdominal fat (i.e., decrease waist circumference) over a period of 6 months. Weight loss will consist of ~75% fat and ~25% lean tissue.
- A deficit of 500–1000 kcal/day produces a weight loss of 70–140 g/day, or 1–2 lbs/week.

During dietary treatment, frequent contact with professional counselors and dieticians promotes increase in weight loss and maintenance. Behavioral treatment *plus* a low-calorie diet is critical for long-term weight loss management. (For the nutrient composition of a low-calorie diet, please see Appendix 3. For additional details on this topic, refer to reference 6.)

Normal Weight

Why Is Counseling Essential?

Primary prevention of overweight must include population-wide efforts among children and adults whose weights are *normal* to encourage them to maintain healthy weight levels. This may be referred to as **anticipatory guidance**. For some, nutrition and physical activity interventions are needed to accomplish maintenance of normal weight. Consider the fact that most overweight/obese patients were at one time normal weight!

Goals of Counseling in Normal-Weight Patients

It takes very little effort to prevent weight gain if consistent activity is maintained while not overeating (see Chapter 7, "Caloric Balance and Expenditure," for details).

- It is much easier to *prevent* increasing BMI; it is harder to take off what has been added.
- The Institute of Medicine recommends 60 minutes of moderate activity (i.e., walking) 5–7 days/week.
- Switching from a 12-ounce cola to water or a diet cola saves 150 kcal.
- The dose-response relationship between BMI and the risk of developing chronic diseases is present even in the healthy range of BMI (Fig. 10–10).

Predictors of Successful Weight Maintenance

Patients who receive and adhere to the following can expect to maintain their weight[7]:

- Physician-mediated physical activity prescription for regular, moderate-intensity physical activity (30 min/day, 5–7days/week)
- Low-calorie diet
- Behavioral therapy and societal support (environments affect populations, e.g., banning smoking in public buildings)
- Continued and frequent contact with healthcare personnel.

Primary Prevention of Weight Gain

Primary prevention is by far the most effective "treatment" to combat weight gain in the first place. The cause of weight gain is caloric imbal-

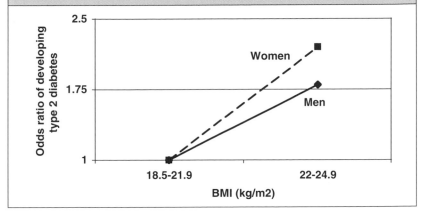

Figure 10–10. Risk of developing diabetes even in the "healthy weight" range of BMI. Men (*solid line*) and women (*dashed line*) with BMIs of 22–24.9 kg/m² had approximately twice the risk of developing type 2 diabetes, compared to those with BMIs of 18.5–21.9 kg/m². (Adapted from Field AE, et al: Impact of overweight on the risk of developing common chronic diseases during a 10-year period. Arch Int Med 161:1581–1586, 2001.)

ance: eating more calories than are expended by physical activity. Thus, primary prevention should target overeating and inertia. Primary prevention will not work unless the patient who is gaining weight is motivated to eat smaller caloric portions at meals. Other approaches include:

- Eating small caloric amounts several times each day
- Saving a portion of a large meal for a second and third meal the next day
- Sharing one large meal with a friend
- Eating calorie-dense foods only on special occasions (once or twice per week)

Being physically active is a wonderful way to maintain a healthy weight. Patients can use stairs instead of elevators/escalators: 1 minute of stair-climbing each day is the caloric equivalent of 1 pound of fat after 1 year for the average-size adult. (Note that about 33% fewer calories are used going *down* stairs. Moreover, the elderly are more likely to trip and fall going down.) Patients can undertake 20 minutes of brisk walking (3 mph) per day: in the average-size adult, this is the caloric equivalent of 10 pounds of fat by the end of 1 year! If time constraints are a problem, the individual might consider buying weights and other exercise equipment for a home gym. Or, since positive reinforcement is available in a group situation, an exercise facility may be best.

It is important to encourage the patient. The individual having trouble maintaining weight or attempting to lose weight can self-motivate, as well, by keeping a chart of body weight. Socializing during physical activity can be fun and adds reinforcement. Sedentary time can be reduced (limit time watching TV).

The American Association of Pediatrics recommends the following guidelines for parents:

- Children should be limited to 1–2 hours with entertainment media per day.
- Remove television sets from children's bedrooms.
- No television viewing for children younger than 2 years of age: encourage interactive pursuits that will promote proper brain development, such as talking, playing, singing, and reading together.

The prevalence of obesity in children and adults has been shown to be directly proportional to the amount of TV watched each day. Moreover, television advertising prompts children to eat fatty and sugary snacks. TV replaces more physically active opportunities. If children spend no more than 2 hours per day in the sedentary activity of TV viewing, they will have less time to snack and will be more likely to engage in spontaneous play.

Secondary Prevention of Obesity

The prevalence of type 2 diabetes in the population increases progressively with increases in body weight. Prevalence is greatest in overweight Hispanics, followed by Afro-Americans; it is lowest in Caucasians. A family history of type 2 diabetes is associated with an increased risk of the disease and requires an aggressive secondary preventive prescription consisting of:

- Monitoring to keep body weight below the 85th percentile for children and adolescents or below 25 kg/m^2 BMI for adults
- Counseling to limit caloric intake if overweight/obese
- Limiting sedentary lifestyle and increasing physical activity.

Tertiary Prevention of Obesity

Adult Tertiary Prevention

Tertiary prevention is medically beneficial, as weight losses of 5–10% of initial body weight can lead to substantial improvement in risk factors for diabetes and heart disease and may allow reduction or discontinuation of medication. However, tertiary prevention only seems to be effective in (at best) 20% of overweight individuals. In successful tertiary treatment interventions, 20% of patients are able to maintain a weight loss of 10% for 1 year, but 80% do *not* maintain this loss. *The 80% failure rate is a very strong argument for primary and secondary prevention.*

Lifestyle Adjustments

Most overweight individuals can effectively lose body weight for short periods (months), but most regain the weight within 1 year. Wing and Hill[7] propose defining successful long-term weight loss maintenance as intentionally losing at least 10% of initial body weight and keeping it off for at least 1 year. In their studies, they achieved > 20% weight loss in overweight/obese persons. In Wing and Hill's National Weight Control Registry (http://www.uchsc.edu/nutrition/nwcr.htm), successful long-term weight loss maintainers averaged a loss of 66 pounds (a drop in 10 BMI units) for an average of 5.5 years. These 3000 individuals were characterized by:

- Long-term, very high motivation to not only lose weight, but to maintain the loss
- Change begun in small steps to reach diet and physical activity goals (see our Small Steps Program in Chapter 8)
- Expenditure of about 400 kcal/day in physical activity, mainly achieved by walking—
    4 miles at a body weight of 154 pounds
    2.6 miles at a bodyweight of 234 pounds
- Consuming an average of 1400 kcal/day (24% from fat)—
    Greater avoidance of fried foods and more substitution of low-fat for high-fat foods than weight regainers
    Eating five meals or snacks/day, which possibly prevents overeating at any one meal
    Eating fast food once/week and at other restaurants 2.5 times/week
- Having been overweight children (67% of successful weight losers)
- Losing weight on their own without any formal weight loss program (60% of total)
- Frequent self-monitoring of body weight and food intake
- A family history of obesity (60% of total).

Pharmacotherapies For Adults

For an excellent summary of the numerous studies elucidating the various pharmacological modalities in the management of obesity, please refer to reference 8 and http://www.niddk.nih.gov/health/nutrit/table.htm.

Medication for obesity should be used only in patients who are at increased medical risk (e.g., hypertension, type 2 DM, coronary artery disease, dyslipidemia) because of their weight; it should not be used for "cosmetic" weight loss. Appropriate weight-loss drugs approved by the FDA for long-term use can augment diet, physical activity, and behavioral

Table 10–3. Summary of Selected Drugs and Their Modes of Action		
Drug	**Action**	**Adverse Effects**
Dexfenfluramine*	Serotonin reuptake inhibitor	Valvular heart disease, primary pulmonary hypertension, neurotoxicity
Fenfluramine*	Serotonin releaser	
Sibutramine	Norepinephrine, dopamine, and serotonin reuptake inhibitor	Increased heart rate and blood pressure
Orlistat	Inhibits pancreatic lipase, decreases fat absorption	Decreased absorption of fat-soluble vitamins, soft stools and anal leakage
* FDA approval withdrawn		

treatment, and should be used *as part of a comprehensive weight loss program*. These drugs should never be used without concomitant lifestyle modification.

If after at least 6 months of low-calorie diets, physical activity, and behavioral treatment, the obese patient has not lost the recommended 1 pound/week, then careful consideration may be given to pharmacotherapy (Table 10–3) for the following subset of patients:

- BMI > 30 kg/m² with no concomitant obesity-related risk factors or diseases
- BMI > 27 kg/m² with concomitant obesity-related risk factors or diseases.

Ephedrine, caffeine, and fluoxetine have also been tested for weight loss, but are not FDA approved for use in the treatment of obesity. Mazindol, phentermine, benzphetamine, and phendimetrazine are approved only for short-term use.

Not every patient responds to drug treatment. If a patient does not lose ~2 kg in the first 4 weeks after initiating treatment, the likelihood of long-term response is very low. If weight is lost in the initial 6 months of treatment, or is maintained after the initial weight loss phase, this should be considered a success, and the drug may be continued. Again, the role of weight loss drugs is to help patients stay on a diet and physical activity plan while losing weight. For more details regarding pharmacotherapies, please refer to reference 6 and http://www.nhlbi.nih.gov/guidelines/obesity/e_txtbk/index.htm.

Surgery

Weight loss surgery (gastric bypass, Roux-en Y, vertical gastric banding) is an option for carefully selected patients with clinically severe obesity (BMI ≥ 40 kg/m² or ≥ 35 kg/m² with comorbid conditions) when less invasive methods of weight loss have failed and the patient is at high risk for obesity-associated morbidity or mortality. These surgical procedures can induce significant weight loss and serve to decrease weight-associated risk factors and comorbidities. Surgery has produced the longest period of sustained weight loss. However, there are several postoperative complications, including malabsorption, vitamin B_{12} deficiency, "dumping syndrome," and cholecystitis. Thus, the risks and benefits need to be carefully evaluated. For more information on surgical therapies, please refer to reference 6 and http://www.nhlbi.nih.gov/guidelines/obesity/e_txtbk/index.htm.

Pediatric Tertiary Prevention

Parenting skills are the foundation for a successful intervention that includes gradual, targeted increases in physical activity and targeted reductions in high-fat, high-calorie foods. Ongoing support for families after the initial weight-management program helps patients maintain their new behaviors. The specific points recommended by an Expert Panel convened by the Maternal and Child Health Bureau, Health Resources and Services Administration, and the Department of Health and Human Services[9] include the following:

- Interventions should begin early.
- The family must be ready for change.
- Clinicians should educate families about medical complications of obesity.
- Clinicians should involve the family and all caregivers in the treatment program.
- Treatment programs should institute permanent changes, not short-term diets or exercise programs aimed at rapid weight loss.
- The family should be taught to monitor eating and activity.
- The treatment program should help the family make small, gradual changes.
- Clinicians should encourage and empathize, not criticize.

According to the Expert Panel, the primary goal of obesity therapy should be healthy eating and physical activity. Details on each of the above bulleted points can be accessed at http://www.pediatrics.org/cgi/content/full/102/3/e29.

Several elements are common to tertiary interventions for childhood obesity.[10] These interventions are family-based, motivating children, adolescents, and parents. If the family is not motivated, behavioral counseling is needed to shift them from the passive/inactive phases of the Stages of Change Model, to the action stages. Be careful to exclude children with eating disorders and their families, because they require specialized treatment. Include meetings with a behavioral specialist in pediatric obesity. Record daily eating and physical activity in "habit books" to assist in behavior change and reinforcements. Teach parents and children to praise specific behavior changes. Establish a point-reward system for children that uses non-monetary rewards (social reinforcement, such as child-parent activities, as rewards). Select rewards that can be maintained after meetings with the behavioral specialist have ended. Urge parents to show model behaviors in front of children. Teach parents how to adjust calories to produce the targeted body weight.

Management Algorithms For Overweight/Obesity

Figure 10–11. Algorithm for adults, to initiate counseling for weight loss and management. (Adapted from http://www.nhlbi.nih.gov/guidelines/obesity/e_txtbk/index.htm.)

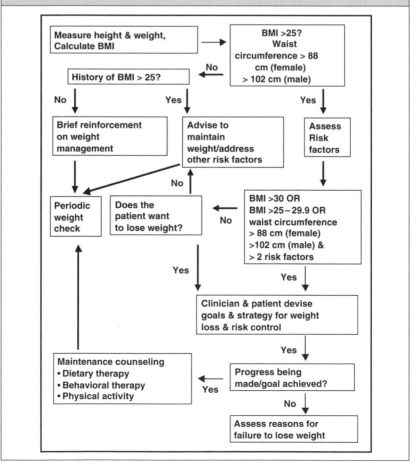

Figure 10–12. Algorithm for children 2–7 years old, to initiate counseling for weight loss and management. *Complications/comorbidities = mild hypertension, dyslipidemias, and insulin resistance. (Adapted from Barlow SE, Dietz WH: Obesity Evaluation and Treatment: Recommendations by an Expert Panel. Pedriatics 102:e29, 1998, also accessible at http://www.pediatrics.org/cgi/content/full/102/3/e29.)

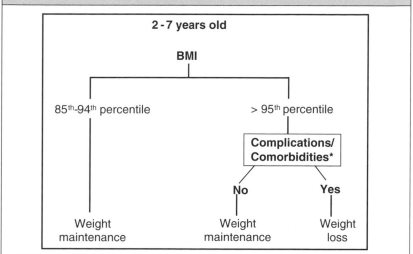

Figure 10–13. Algorithm for children ≥ 7 years old, to initiate counseling for weight loss and management. *Complications/comorbidities = mild hypertension, dyslipidemias, and insulin resistance. (Adapted from Barlow SE, Dietz WH: Obesity Evaluation and Treatment: Recommendations by an Expert Panel. Pedriatics 102:e29, 1998, also accessible at http://www.pediatrics.org/cgi/content/full/102/3/e29.)

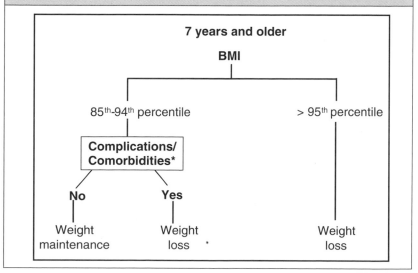

Children/adolescents qualifying for additional evaluation and treatment:

- Children < 2 years of age with a BMI > 95th percentile
- BMI ≥ 85th percentile with complications/comorbidities of obesity
- BMI ≥ 95th percentile, with or without complications/comorbidities of obesity
- Patients with acute complications, such as pseudotumor cerebri, severe hypertension, sleep apnea, obesity hypoventilation syndrome, orthopedic disorders, or gallbladder disease
- Rare causes of obesity, including genetic syndromes, endocrinologic diseases, and psychologic disorders.

Key Points

∞ Primary prevention counseling is a key strategy because obesity is a *national public health concern.*

∞ Preventing weight gain in the first place, especially in the lower socioeconomic strata and uninsured groups, would have a tremendous public health impact, as well as a substantial benefit on national governmental budgets.

∞ There is compelling evidence in the literature to suggest that physician-mediated counseling *is effective* in making people want to lose weight.

∞ Such counseling *does help* to markedly decrease the incidence of obesity-associated conditions (e.g., type 2 diabetes, cardiovascular disease).

Suggested Reading

1. Calle EE, Thun MJ, Petrelli JM, et al. Body-mass index and mortality in a prospective cohort of U.S. adults. New Engl J Med 341:1097–1105, 1999.
2. Field AE, et al. Impact of overweight on the risk of developing common chronic diseases during a 10-year period. Arch Intern Med 161:1581–1586, 2001.
3. Hu FB, Sigal RJ, Rich-Edwards JW, et al. Walking compared with vigorous physical activity and risk of type 2 diabetes in women: A prospective study. JAMA 282: 1433–1439, 1999.
4. Manson JE, Hu FB, Rich-Edwards JW, et al. A prospective study of walking as compared with vigorous exercise in the prevention of coronary heart disease in women. New Engl J Med 341: 650–658, 1999.
5. Hu FB, Stampfer MJ, Colditz GA, et al. Physical activity and risk of stroke in women. JAMA 283: 2961–2967, 2000.
6. Bessesen, Kushner. Obesity. Philadelphia, Hanley & Belfus, 2001.
7. Wing RR, Hill JO. Successful weight loss maintenance. Annu Rev Nutr 21:323–341, 2001.

8. National Task Force on the Prevention and Treatment of Obesity. Long-term pharmacotherapy in the management of obesity. JAMA 276:1907–1915, 1996.

9. Barlow SE, Dietz WH Obesity Evaluation and Treatment: Recommendations by an Expert Panel. Pedriatics 102:e29, 1998, also accessible at http://www.pediatrics.org/cgi/content/full/102/3/e29)

10. Epstein LH, Roemmich JN, Raynor HA. Behavioral therapy in the treatment of pediatric obesity. Pediatr Clin North Am 48:981–993, 2001.

11. Kimm SY, Glynn NW, Kriska AM, et al. Decline in physical activity in black girls and white girls during adolescence. New Engl J Med 347: 709–715, 2002.

12. Rippe JM, McInnis KJ, Melanson KJ. Physician involvement in the management of obesity as a primary medical condition. Obes Res Suppl 4: 302S–311S, 2001.

Promotion of Routine Daily Physical Activity

Although many benefits of physical activity have been demonstrated in large multi-center epidemiological and laboratory studies (see Chapter 6 for details), the major challenge to the clinician is translating these beneficial findings to the practical realm of patient encouragement and promotion of daily physical activity. Indeed, this challenge forms the core of the *Healthy People 2010* objectives[1]: to increase the amount of moderate or vigorous physical activity performed by people in all population subgroups, and to increase the opportunities for physical activity by creating and enhancing access to places and facilities where people can be physically active (Table 11–1). This chapter discusses interventions

Table 11–1.   Healthy People 2010: Selected Objectives For Increasing Physical Activity

Activity (Or Lack Thereof)	Population Assessed	Percentage of Population	
		Baseline*	2010 Goal
No leisure time physical activity	Adult	40% (1997)	Reduce to 20%
At least 30 min moderate physical activity (preferably daily)	Adult	15% (1997)	Increase to 30%
Trips of < 1 mile by walking	Adults	17% (1995)	Increase to 25%
Trips of < 5 miles by bicycling	Adults	0.6% (1995)	Increase to 2%
Vigorous physical activity	Adult	23% (1997)	Increase to 30%
promoting development and maintenance of cardiorespiratory fitness > 3 days/wk for 20 min/session	Adolescents	65% (1997)	Increase to 85%
Daily school physical education	Adolescents	29% (1999)	Increase to 50%
View television < 2 hr on a school day	Adolescents	57% (1999)	Increase to 75%

*Years indicate when the data was analyzed to establish baseline estimates. Some of the estimates are age-adjusted to the year 2000 standard population.
Adapted from U.S. Dept of Health and Human Services: *Healthy People 2010,* conference edition. Washington DC, U.S. Department of Health and Human Services, 2000.

that have proved effective in reaching these objectives, both at the individual and community levels.

Individual-Oriented Promotion

Personal Energy Plan: This is a 12-week, self-directed worksite program to promote healthy eating and moderate physical activity among employees. The program materials include workbooks for healthy eating and physical activity targeting employees based on their readiness to change. A coordinator's kit, promotional brochures, and posters are also included. For details, please visit http://www.cdc.gov/nccdphp/dnpa/pep.htm.

Physical activity tips: A CDC website provides information to individuals who wish to add physical activity to their daily routines at home, work, and elsewhere. For details, please see http://www.cdc.gov/nccdphp/dnpa/phys_act.htm.

Physical Activity Evaluation Handbook: This CDC resource outlines six basic steps to evaluate a physical activity program and illustrates each step with examples. Appendices provide information about physical activity indicators, practical case studies, and additional evaluation resources. The website contains both PDF and HTML files of the Physical Activity Handbook, as well as an address to which to write for a copy. See http://www.cdc.gov/nccdphp/dnpa/physical/handbook/index.htm.

Choose to Move: A self-paced, 12-week physical activity program for women developed by the American Heart Association (http://www.choosetomove.org/about.html). Men are encouraged to participate as well! Skills learned include staying active and motivated. The program emphasizes that while the participant may stop and start again, the important thing is to keep moving. The goal is to accumulate 30 min/day of moderately intense physical activity on 5 or more days a week. A recently published study[2] showed that among the participants who completed the 12-week program, the percentage who reported being active (at least moderate exercise $\geq$ 5 times per week or $\geq$ 2 hours per week for the past 1 to 6 months) increased from 32% at baseline to 67% at the program's end ($P = .001$). In addition, program participants also significantly reduced their consumption of high-fat foods and increased their knowledge and awareness of cardiovascular disease risk and symptoms. This program provides an important model of a population-based, targeted, low-cost self-help program for public health, voluntary, and other health organizations.

INTERVENT: Individual-based lifestyle and behavior modification program, empowering participants to make meaningful changes, including increased physical activity, correct nutrition, and weight management (http://interventusa.com). The program helps participants reduce their risk for cardiovascular disease and other potentially preventable chronic illnesses. A recently published study using INTERVENT in high-risk cardiac patients[3] demonstrated a favorable risk reduction in many of the cardiac risk factors, including significant (p < 0.05) reduction in systolic (−16 mmHg) and diastolic (−18 mmHg) pressures, total cholesterol (−75 mg/dL), LDL-cholesterol (−61 mg/dL), triglycerides (−82 mg/dL), and significantly (p < 0.05) increased HDL-cholesterol (+ 11 mg/dL). Interestingly, patients with the worst coronary risk factor profiles at baseline demonstrated the greatest improvements after the program.

10,000 Steps: Physical activity studies show that wearing a pedometer is effective in tracking daily activity, and therefore is a powerful physical activity motivator. Participants wore the Digiwalker pedometer on their belt or waistband to determine their current level of activity; for most it was 3000–5000 steps/day. Then with the feedback the pedometer provided, they developed and implemented strategies to gradually reach the goal of at least 10,000 steps per day (the equivalent of about 5 miles), which burns 2000–3500 extra kcal/week. Results include lower body fat, improved blood pressure, and increased cardiorespiratory fitness. For weight loss, 12,000–15,000 steps/day would be needed. Further details can be obtained at http://www.digiwalker.com.

Population-Based Promotion

Several interventional strategies have been proposed and evaluated in a systematic review by Kahn, et al[4] and Eden, et al.[5] The formal recommendations of the Task Force on Community Preventive Services[6] specifically address the effectiveness of community-based programs that target groups rather than individual patients (Table 11–2). A number of other interventions have been effective in promoting physical activity:

Community-wide campaigns (policy interventions and partnership organizations): Legislation establishing financial incentives for organizations and communities to provide access to gyms/exercise programs; use of programs such as Planned Approach To Community Health (PATCH) and Physical Activity Risk Reduction (PARR)

Schools: Changes in school-based physical education programs and curricula, emphasizing skill-oriented interventions and health education classes

Changing the physical environment: Increasing activity opportunities by improved access to places to undertake physical activity (parks, recreational facilities, neighborhood play areas); safe, lighted walking paths

Program links: Linking individual-based behavior change programs to community-based physical activity and fitness programs to provide

TABLE 11–2. Recommendations of the Task Force on Community Preventive Services—Interventions To Increase Physical Activity

Intervention	Recommendation*
Informational Approaches to Increasing Physical Activity	
Community-wide campaigns	Strongly recommended
• Increased the percentage of people who are active, their estimated energy expenditure, and their activity levels.	
• Resulted in a 5% increase in the proportion of people who are physically active and a 16% increase in energy expenditure.	
• Effective in both rural and urban communities and among different ethnic and socioeconomic groups.	
• Improved the health of communities by developing or strengthening social networks and by improving community members' sense of cohesion and collective ability to bring about change.	
"Point-of-decision" prompts to encourage stair use	Recommended
• More people used the stairs (increased stair use from a baseline of ~12% to ~54%) when these signs were posted.	
• This intervention was shown to be effective in a variety of settings including train, subway, and bus stations, shopping malls, and university libraries and in a variety of population subgroups including men and women, both obese and not obese.	
• Tailoring the prompts to describe specific benefits or to appeal to specific populations may increase the intervention's effectiveness. For example, in one study, obese people used the stairs more if the signs linked stair use to weight loss rather than to general health benefits.	
Classroom-based health education focused on information provision	Insufficient evidence**
Mass media campaigns	Insufficient evidence**
Behavioral and Social Approaches to Increasing Physical Activity	
School-based physical education	Strongly recommended
• Overall, students' physical fitness improved, including increases in the (1) number of minutes spent in moderate or vigorous physical activity, (2) percentage of class time spent in moderate or vigorous physical activity, and/or (3) intensity level of physical activity during class.	
• Median estimates suggest that modifying school PE curricula as recommended will result in an 8% increase in aerobic fitness among school-aged children; was effective across diverse racial, ethnic, and socioeconomic groups, among boys and girls, elementary- and high-school students, and in urban and rural settings.	
• Further, having students attend school PE classes was *not* found to harm academic performance.	

(continued)

TABLE 11–2. Recommendations of the Task Force on Community Preventive Services—Interventions To Increase Physical Activity *(Continued)*

Intervention	Recommendation*
Social support interventions in community settings • Effective in getting people to be more physically active, as measured by various indicators (e.g., blocks walked or flights of stairs climbed daily, frequency of attending exercise sessions, or minutes spent in physical activity). • Median estimates suggested a 44% increase in time spent being physically active and a 20% increase in the frequency of physical activity. • Improved participants' fitness levels, lowered their percentage of body fat, increased their knowledge about exercise, and improved their confidence in their ability to exercise. • Effective in various settings including communities, worksites, and universities, among men and women, adults of different ages, and both sedentary people and those who were already active.	Strongly recommended
Individually-adapted health behavior change programs • Resulted in a 35% increase in the amount of time people spend being physically active and a 64% increase in energy expenditure. Also, the percentage of people starting exercise programs and the frequency of physical activity increased. • Effective among both men and women and in a variety of settings, including communities, worksites, and schools.	Strongly recommended
Classroom-based health education focused on reducing television viewing and video game playing	Insufficient evidence**
College-age health education and physical education	Insufficient evidence**
Family-based social support	Insufficient evidence**
Environmental and Policy Approaches to Increasing Physical Activity	
Creation of, or enhanced access to, places for physical activity; combined with informational outreach activities • Resulted in a 25% increase in the number of persons who exercise at least 3 times a week. • Most of the studies also reported weight losses or decreases in body fat among program participants. • Effective among both men and women and in various settings, including industrial plants, universities, federal agencies, and low-income communities.	Strongly recommended
Transportation policy and infrastructure changes to promote non-motorized transit • One set of barriers is the way roads, highways, sidewalks, bike paths, suburban developments, and community infrastructures are built. • Planning and zoning commissions/policy-makers are not sufficiently aware of the direct impact that zoning and land use planning has on promoting a physically active population.	Awaiting formal recommendations

(continued)

TABLE 11–2. Recommendations of the Task Force on Community Preventive Services—Interventions To Increase Physical Activity *(Continued)*	
Intervention	**Recommendation***
Urban planning approaches—zoning and land use	Awaiting formal recommendations

* Strongly recommended = strong evidence that the intervention is effective; Recommended = adequate evidence that the intervention is effective. The strength of evidence is determined by the number of studies with suitable study designs and acceptable quality of execution, according to the methods employed in developing *The Community Guide.*[6]
** A determination of insufficient evidence should not be confused with evidence of ineffectiveness. It only means that the Task Force was unable to issue a recommendation due to a lack of good-quality studies or due to conflicting evidence of effectiveness in the studies reviewed. A determination of insufficient evidence assists in identifying (a) areas of uncertainty regarding an intervention's effectiveness, and (b) gaps in the evidence where future prevention research is needed. *In contrast, evidence of ineffectiveness leads to a recommendation that the intervention not be used.*

behavioral reinforcements; use of incentives to change physical activity behavior

Volunteer groups: Volunteers who deliver physical activity messages at community sites, worksites, schools; offer physical activity courses and health promotion classes

Social mechanisms: Use of group settings to enhance social support (designating walking partners, family-based programs, faith-based social support, physical activity clubs)

Provider training: To change knowledge, attitudes, and behavior about physical activity screening and promotion; Physician-based Assessment and Counseling for Exercise (PACE), and Physically Active for Life (PAL) programs; physicians encouraged to work in their communities to establish local health councils and promote physical activity (think globally, act locally).

Partnership For Prevention: A national nonprofit organization dedicated to preventing and promoting health. Information on community-based promotion of physical activity in the elderly can be accessed at http://www.prevent.org.

Centers for Disease Control Programs

Active Community Environments: A CDC-sponsored initiative to promote walking, bicycling, and the development of accessible recreational facilities (http://www.cdc.gov/nccdphp/dnpa/aces.htm)

Kids Walk-To-School: Developed by the CDC's Nutrition and Physical Activity Program to support the national goal of better health through physical activity (http://www.cdc.gov/nccdphp/dnpa/kidswalk/index.htm). This is a community-based program that aims to increase opportunities for daily physical activity by encouraging children to walk to and from school in groups accompanied by adults.

Strategies promoting lifelong exercise: Better health for young people through physical activity and sports. This report from the Secretary of Health and Human Services and the Secretary of Education, recently released by the White House, outlines 10 strategies to promote health and reduce obesity through lifelong participation in enjoyable and safe physical activity and sports (http://www.cdc.gov/nccdphp/dash/presphysactrpt/index.htm).

Guide to Community Preventive Services: Effective population-level strategies to promote physical activity; reports evidence-based recommendations (http://www.cdc.gov/nccdphp/dnpa/physical/recommendations.htm).

Recommendations of the Task Force on Community Preventive Services

The Task Force on Community Preventive Services has issued a list of recommended interventions to increase physical activity (Table 11–2).[6] The Task Force was supported by the Physical Activity Systematic Review Team. Each recommendation is based on the strength of the evidence of effectiveness found during systematic reviews. Decision-makers should consider these evidence-based recommendations and local needs, goals, and constraints when choosing appropriate interventions. Details of the Task Force's recommendations are available at http://www.thecommunityguide.org/physical_f1.html.

These interventions are appropriate for those who are interested in or responsible for planning, selecting, funding, and/or implementing community, policy, and public health interventions to increase people's physical activity levels. They fall into three broad categories:

1. Informational approaches—provide people with information that will motivate and enable them to change their behavior (e.g., increase their physical activity level) and maintain that change over time

2. Behavioral and social approaches—teach people behavioral management skills necessary for the successful adoption and maintenance of behavior change, and on structuring social environments to provide support for behavioral change

3. Environmental and policy approaches—change the structure of the physical and organizational environments to provide safe, attractive, and convenient places for physical activity, through the development of public policy, creation of supportive environments, and strengthening of community action

The Task Force based its findings on the results of a systematic, evidence-based analysis of the scientific literature. For each intervention, the Task Force searched for published evidence and conducted a standardized review of each study identified. A summary of the evidence relating to effectiveness, possible harms, barriers to implementation, and cost-effectiveness was then prepared. Also addressed was the range of settings and populations in which the intervention was effective. Task Force recommendations are based primarily on the evidence of *effectiveness* of an intervention. Following this approach, the Task Force *strongly recommends* five interventions and *recommends* one intervention to increase physical activity levels (see Table 11–2). The Task Force supports use of both "strongly recommended" and "recommended" interventions.

Promotion of Physical Activity For Specific Age Groups

Pediatric Population

TABLE 11–3. Methods Physicians Can Use to Promote Physical Activity in Children/Adolescents		
Objective	**Target**	**Strategy**
Incorporate physical activity counseling into medical practice	Children, parents, and physicians	Ask about physical activity patterns, encourage parents to be more active, and recommend activities specific to the child's age, family circumstances, and environment.
Universal participation in increased physical activity	All children, including those who are clumsy, overweight, or handicapped	For older children, emphasize sports in which they can participate all their life. De-emphasize the competitive and achievement-oriented nature of sports programs; focus on participation and teamwork. Encourage an active lifestyle at a young age.
Improve children's access to physical activity programs	Schools, media, and local, state, and national government	Improve physical education programs in schools and daycare; encourage the maintenance of high-quality and safe public play spaces; and promote life-long participation in sports and the benefits of a physically active lifestyle.
Adapted from Williams, CL, Hayman, LL, Daniels, SR, et al: Cardiovascular Health in Childhood: A Statement for Health Professionals From the Committee on Atherosclerosis, Hypertension, and Obesity in the Young (AHOY) of the Council on Cardiovascular Disease in the Young, American Heart Association. Circulation 106: 143–160, 2002.		

Other promotional strategies:
- Physical activity during school recesses

- Encouragement of lifetime physical activity in physical education classes
- Teaching in schools about the biological and medical basis by which physical inactivity increases the risk of chronic health conditions
- Training students how to count calories used walking and climbing stairs
- Teaching and encouraging healthy nutrition habits by minimizing junk foods in school cafeterias
- Recreational sports for those students whose skills do not allow them to compete on interscholastic athletic teams
- Education of parents on how to maintain healthy behaviors for the entire family
- Safe and friendly communities for physical activity (e.g., safe paths to walk or cycle to school, opening of school gyms for after-hours physical activities).

Physician advocacy groups can be powerful in effecting the above-listed goals. There are other projects they can undertake for the primary prevention of pediatric obesity, as well. Remember that the cost and effort to convince all adults to become physically active again after becoming inactive is much greater than the cost of preventing children/adolescents from becoming physically inactive in the first place.

- Elimination of TV advertisements promoting junk foods
- Limitations on TV watching—no TV in the bedrooms of preschoolers
- Neighborhood eateries offering fewer calorie-dense foods and in smaller portions
- End to street crime (e.g., Walkers on Watch, tied in with Neighborhood Crime Watch programs)
- Lobby school boards for:
  (1) Biology curriculum to include instruction on how physical inactivity decreases functional capacity, lessens the ability to withstand stress to organ systems, and starts the progression of chronic diseases
  (2) Health curriculum to instruct on the epidemiology of chronic diseases caused by a sedentary lifestyle
  (3) Physical education classes to provide equality of instruction and reinforce enjoyment of physical activity.

Adults and the Elderly Population

It has been shown that strength of physicians' advice is significantly correlated with the likelihood of adopting increased physical activity in older patients.[8] Therefore, every possible effort must be made to counsel increased physical activity. Some of the approaches include:

- Family play and outings; neighborhood sidewalks, safe parks in urban areas, school gyms, and community recreational buildings
- Employer encouragement of a minimum of 30 minutes of physical activity each day, as part of health coverage benefits
- Lobbying of legislators, corporate heads, and community leaders to support a physically active America
- Inclusion of physical activity at social gatherings
- For seniors, free access to strength training equipment and recreational facilities; education about the effects of a sedentary lifestyle on vitality, quality of life, and ability to perform tasks of daily living.

Many patients need close guidance, support, and encouragement to increase, nurture, and sustain the physical activity behavior. Some people, even if they want to become active, don't know how to go about it, or they may have fears of exercise (propagated by news media sensationalizing when a jogger dies for example) or distasteful memories of physical activities. Physician-mediated advice is highly effective in *initiating* physical activity, but advocating sustained physical activity for the long term is labor-intensive, and often cannot be done by giving advice in isolation. Therefore, physicians should use allied healthcare professionals (e.g., clinical exercise physiologists, nutritionists, competent personal trainers), when possible, to work with their patients as they adopt sustained physical activity. The American College of Sports Medicine offers several programs, including WellCoaches (www.wellcoach.com), that individuals can access for a health enhancement program. For additional details regarding the promotion of increased physical activity in the elderly, especially in community-wide efforts, please refer to http://www.prevent.org (see reference 9).

Economic Considerations

Cost can be used as a weapon to fight for a change to a more physically active society. For example, Colditz (10) suggested that focused strategies to increase the level of physical activity will likely produce substantial benefits through reduced healthcare costs and indirect costs, and gains in quality of life. One crucial target is the 70% of the U.S. population who are now sedentary. However, the cost weapon has not been widely employed. Fries et al (11) wrote: "Advocates of health promotion have themselves caused delays, first by not making cost reduction a primary goal, and second by neglecting rigorous economic evaluation."

It is our belief that there now exists sufficient and rather convincing cost-of-illness data (a minimum of $150 billion in annual direct and indirect costs for physical inactivity[12]) to demand immediate cost-effectiveness studies. These studies would likely justify the promotion of moderate-intensity physical activity to reduce healthcare expenditures.

Media Campaigns

The Task Force On Community Preventive Services could not recommend mass media campaigns (due to insufficient evidence; see Table 11–2) for dissemination of public information and social marketing. Thus, studies are needed to explore and formally assess the effectiveness of the following campaigns:

1. Improving the public's knowledge and attitudes about benefits of and opportunities for physical activity

2. Changing social norms about desirability or need for physical activity

3. Creating a demand for increased opportunities to undertake physical activity.

As the Task Force noted, "insufficient evidence" does *not* mean mass media campaigns are ineffective. We recommend trying dissemination of information to the general public via various formats and media as a means for change. Educating the general public about the existence of a large body of scientific evidence supporting the many positive benefits of a physically active lifestyle in promoting good health empowers them to become proactive. Such active individual involvement could effect a fundamental shift in the way society thinks about the ongoing war on modern chronic diseases.

Broader Programs

The **National Coalition for the Promotion of Physical Activity** (http://www.ncppa.org) champions three specific goals that require policy change:

1. Reverse unintended barriers to physical activity for populations with low rates of activity.

2. Increase the adoption of activity-friendly community models.

3. Promote incentives for physical activity behaviors in worksite, community, and school settings.

The **Improved Nutrition and Physical Activity Act** (IMPACT) provides grants to train primary care physicians and other healthcare professionals in identifying, treating, and preventing obesity and aiding individuals who are overweight. It also offers local grants for city, county, tribe, or state to increase physical activity and improve nutrition in all age groups. Local educational grants allow development of school-based curriculums or programs that focus on healthy lifestyles, including balanced dietary patterns to prevent becoming overweight or obese. The Act also encompasses youth media campaigns designed to change children's health behaviors.

The **Statement from the 2002 National Governor's Conference** indicates that states are addressing the obesity epidemic with innovative food and physical activity policies/standards, healthy community design, public education, healthcare systems, and tax strategies. The following points are also made:

- Obesity is not just a matter of personal health—it's a costly and deadly public health concern that affects economic productivity, state budgets, and personal and family well being.
- Thirteen percent of children and adolescents are now overweight or obese, which represents more than a doubling in the last 30 years. Minority groups and those with less education and lower income are much more likely to be overweight and obese.
- Nearly 30% of African-American adults and 23 of Hispanic adults are obese. One in five Hispanic and African-American children are overweight.
- There has been a 10-fold increase in the number of children with adult-onset diabetes in the last 5 years. The results of this ongoing problem are additional absence from work and school, lost productivity, and higher healthcare costs.
- At-risk and overweight children increasingly suffer from depression, anxiety, social angst, diabetes, and other health problems, and are more likely to grow up to be obese adults.
- States are paying heavily for obesity and its care—currently, 4 million obese children are Medicaid beneficiaries, and an unknown number of adult Medicaid beneficiaries are obese.

There is much work to be done to significantly improve health and the associated healthcare costs. Fortunately, states are leading the way in addressing this problem. Much of the death, disease, and disability associated with obesity can be prevented through state actions to increase physical activity, promote better diet, and improve prevention and treatment available through healthcare systems.

Researchers Against Inactivity-Related Diseases (www.endseds.org) has three basic goals: (1) to encourage NIH to develop a strategic plan for research to counter inactivity-related disorders, (2) to encourage the Center for Scientific Review at NIH to ensure that research proposals about inactivity-related diseases receive a fair review (at least 30% of peer reviewers at initial grant review meetings should have published papers on physical activity), and (3) to reverse the Center for Scientific Review's position that physical *in*activity does not cut across organ systems.

Key Points

co Pysicians can use their positions to promote physical activity in the community. For example, some doctors act as team physicians and influence sports practices.

co Team physicians, healthcare professionals, and coaches should lead the way and be role models by advocating healthy lifestyle behaviors.

co Healthcare professionals can provide school boards with the health reasons for offering recesses, physical education classes, after-hours recreation facilities, and play areas, and for limiting the availability of unhealthy snack-foods in school settings.

co Healthcare professionals can promote the availability of equipment and trainers for older individuals to delay the onset of physical frailty.

co The scientific and healthcare community has successfully prevented and eradicated many infectious and nutritional diseases (e.g., small pox, scurvy). Therefore, the same result should be possible for chronic debilitating diseases such as diabetes, obesity, and heart disease by employing primary prevention modalities—including physical activity.

Suggested Reading

1. U.S. Dept of Health and Human Services. Healthy People 2010, conference edition. Washington DC, U.S. Dept of Health and Human Services, 2000.

2. Koffman DM, et al. An evaluation of Choose To Move 1999: An American Heart Association physical activity program for women. Arch Intern Med161: 2193–2199, 2001.

3. Franklin B, et al. Effects of a contemporary, exercise-based rehabilitation and cardiovascular risk-reduction program on coronary patients with abnormal baseline risk factors. Chest 122: 338–343, 2002.

4. Kahn EB, Ramsey LT, Brownson RC, et al, and the Task Force on Community Preventive Services. The effectiveness of interventions to increase physical activity: A systematic review. Am J Prev Med 22(4s): 73–107, 2002.

5. Eden KB, et al. Does counseling by clinicians improve physical activity? A summary of the evidence from the U.S. Preventive Services Task Force. Ann Intern Med 137: 208–215, 2002.

6. Recommendations to increase physical activity in communities. Am J Prev Med 22(4 Suppl): 67–72, 2002. Can also be accessed at http://www.thecommunityguide.org

7. Williams CL, Hayman LL, Daniels SR, et al. Cardiovascular Health in Childhood: A Statement for Health Professionals From the Committee on Atherosclerosis, Hypertension, and Obesity in the Young (AHOY) of the Council on Cardiovascular Disease in the Young, American Heart Association. Circulation 106: 143–160, 2002.

8. Ades PA, Waldmann M, McCann W, Wever SO. Predictors of cardiac rehabilitation participation in older coronary patients. Arch Intern Med 152: 1033–1035, 1992.

9. Creating communities for active aging. Published online at http://www.prevent.org/Winword/CCFAA.pdf though the Partnership for prevention organization.

10. Colditz GA. Economic costs of obesity and inactivity. Med. Sci. Sports Exerc 31: S663-S667, 1999.

11. Fries JF, Koop CE., Beadle CE, et al, and the Health Project Consortium. Reducing health care costs by reducing the need and demand for medical services. New Engl J Med 329: 321–325, 1993.

12. Pratt M, Macera CA, Wang G. Higher direct medical costs associated with physical inactivity. Physician Sportsmed 28: 63–70, 2000.

SECTION III
The Biological Basis For Chronic Diseases Caused By Physical Inactivity

chapter
12

Health Consequences of Physical Inactivity

Metabolic Syndrome and Insulin Resistance/ Hyperinsulinemia

Metabolic Syndrome

The Executive Summary of the Third Report of the National Cholesterol Education Program (NCEP) Expert Panel on Detection, Evaluation, and Treatment of High Blood Cholesterol in Adults (Adult Treatment Panel III [ATPIII]) defines the metabolic syndrome as comprising three of five lipid and nonlipid risk factors of metabolic origin (Table 12–1)[1]. Physical activity diminishes the magnitude of all five risk factors!

TABLE 12–1. Metabolic Syndrome: Cluster of Abnormalities		
Components of the Metabolic Syndrome	Change With Physical *In*activity	Change With Physical Activity
Large abdominal circumference: Women > 35 inches Men > 40 inches	Increases	Decreases
Hypertriglycidemia: > 150 mg/dL	Increases	Decreases
Low HDL: Women < 50 mg/dL Men < 40 mg/dL	Decreases	Increases
High blood pressure: > 130/85 mmHg	Increases	Decreases
High fasting blood glucose: > 110 mg/dL	Increases	Decreases

Adapted from the Expert Panel on Detection, Evaluation, and Treatment of High Blood Cholesterol in Adults. Executive Summary of the Third Report of the National Cholesterol Education Program (NCEP) Expert Panel on Detection, Evaluation, and Treatment of High Blood Cholesterol in Adults (Adult Treatment Panel III). JAMA 285:2486, 2002.

These five criteria for the metabolic syndrome are commonly measured in physical exams, and thus are readily available to the clinician. The physician should consider all five together in making the diagnosis, rather than each separately. When three or more cluster in a patient, the risk for coronary heart disease (CHD) is much higher than if the patient had a single abnormality. One of the key benefits in using the **cluster of metabolic abnormalities** for diagnosis is the recognition that CHD is not limited to hypercholesterolemia.[2] Paying attention to whether there is a clustering of the five abnormal values will improve the odds that the appropriate therapeutic decision is made.

Interestingly, the metabolic syndrome does not include the abnormality of insulin resistance. Thus, the presence or absence of insulin resistance is the defining difference between the metabolic syndrome and the insulin resistance syndrome. Three of the five factors in the metabolic syndrome are poorly related to insulin resistance:

- While fasting blood glucose > 110 mg/dL is highly predictive of insulin resistance/hyperinsulinemia, fasting blood glucose *per se* is not a sensitive indicator because the vast majority of insulin-resistant/hyperinsulinemic patients have a fasting glucose concentration < 110 mg/dL.[2]
- Only 25% of obese individuals are insulin resistant.[2]
- Only 50% of hypertensive patients are insulin resistant.[2]

Hence, to accurately identify patients who are insulin resistant, a broader classification of the clustered metabolic abnormalities must be considered.

Insulin Resistance Syndrome

Even if a patient's measured fasting blood glucose concentration is < 110 mg/dL and abdominal circumference is < 35 inches, you cannot conclusively conclude that the patient has no insulin resistance (IR) because, as noted above, many IR patients have normal fasting glucose and are not obese. The two metabolic syndrome criteria most highly correlated with IR/hyperinsulinemia are abnormal plasma triglycerides and HDL-C concentrations.[2] Thus, the significance of identifying patients at risk for IR beyond just the standard metabolic syndrome is that the clustering of some of the abnormalities associated with IR is much more extensive, with a wider array of disorders, including abnormalities in uric aid metabolism and derangements in endothelial, hematologic, and neuroendocrine function. This abnormal metabolic clustering of parameters is termed the insulin resistance syndrome (Table 12–2).

The risk of CHD, type 2 diabetes, and hypertension (~50% of patients with hypertension are insulin resistant) is markedly increased with clustering of any of the abnormalities associated with the IR syndrome. Phys-

TABLE 12–2. Insulin Resistance Syndrome: Cluster of Abnormalities		
Abnormalities Associated With Insulin Resistance/Hyperinsulinemia	**Change With Physical Inactivity**	**Change With Physical Activity**
Glucose intolerance		
• Impaired fasting glucose	Raises	Lowers
• Impaired glucose tolerance	Raises	Lowers
Abnormal uric acid metabolism		
• Increased plasma uric acid concentration	Unknown	Lowers
• Decreased renal uric acid clearance	ND	ND
Dyslipidemia		
• Increased fasting TG	Increases more	Slight decrease
• Decreased fasting HDL-C	Decreases more	Increases HDL-C 5%
• Increased fasting LDL	Increases more	Decrease or no change
• Increases postprandial lipemia	Increases greatly	Major lowering
Hemodynamic		
• Increased sympathetic nervous system activity	Increases	Large decreases
• Increased BP (50% of patients w/hypertension are insulin resistant)	Small, but clinically significant rise	Small, but clinically significant fall
Hemostatic		
• Increased plasminogen activator inhibitor 1	Unknown	Only strenuous exercise decreases
• Increased fibrinogen	ND	Sometimes lowered in randomized clinical trial
Endothelial dysfunction		
• Increased mononuclear cell adhesion	Increases more	Decreases
• Increased plasma concentration of CADs	ND	ND
• Decreased endothelial-dependent vasodilatation	Major decline	Major increase
Reproductive		
• Polycystic ovary syndrome	Unknown	Lowers incidence

CADs = cellular adhesion molecules, ND = not determined
Adapted from Reaven G. Metabolic syndrome: Pathophysiology and implications for management of cardiovascular disease. Circulation 106:286–288, 2002.

ical activity/inactivity also affects each of the parameters associated with the IR syndrome.

Note that most of the criteria for the IR syndrome, unlike those for the metabolic syndrome, are *not* commonly measured in physical exams. This is a crucial difference, underscoring the importance of clinically recognizing the abnormalities associated with the IR syndrome. The presence of even one of these features indicates that the patient may have some of the other abnormalities as well, since they tend to occur in clusters. The IR syndrome ultimately places these patients at a very high risk for morbid chronic diseases.

Insulin resistance is not a disease entity by itself. However, the more insulin resistant a patient is, the more likely he or she is to have one or more of the other abnormalities (see Table 12–2). Furthermore, not all insulin-resistant patients develop every abnormality, nor are the abnormalities solely regulated by insulin resistance/hyperinsulinemia. Interestingly, abdominal obesity is *not* a manifestation of the IR syndrome, and only 25% of obese individuals are insulin resistant.

Therapeutic Implications

As excess adiposity and physical inactivity are the major lifestyle variables that have an untoward effect on insulin action, weight loss and increased physical activity, when appropriately initiated, will enhance insulin sensitivity and decrease the associated CHD risk factors. Regardless of how we ultimately categorize these clusters, the bottom line is that physical inactivity increases the prevalence of both the metabolic syndrome and the insulin resistance syndrome, and physical activity can be used as primary and secondary prevention.

Prevalence of the Metabolic/Insulin Resistance Syndrome

The prevalence of metabolic syndrome increases with age (Fig. 12–1). Approximately 22% of U.S. adults (56 million) have this syndrome, and its prevalence continues to increase, with nearly 45% of individuals having the disorder by their seventh decade. Prevalence also increases as cardiovascular fitness decreases, and risk is 5- and 10-fold higher in the "least fit" compared to "most fit" (Fig. 12–2). In fact, physical inactivity is a strong predictor for the development of the metabolic syndrome.

Recent epidemiological data from Finland[5] shows that subjects engaging in > 3 hr/wk of moderate-intensity leisure-time physical activity were *half as likely* as sedentary subjects to have the metabolic syndrome. Indeed, men in the upper third of aerobic fitness (those who undertook > 3 hr/wk of *vigorous* activity) were 75% *less likely* than unfit men to develop the disorder. The subjects were 612 middle-aged men who started the study without the metabolic syndrome; they were followed prospectively, and the effects of moderate and vigorous physical activity were assessed over a 4-year period and compared to a subgroup of men who remained sedentary.

The significance of this study lies in the fact that this is the first prospective study to show a direct association of physical inactivity with

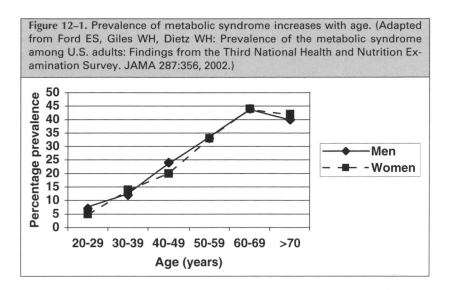

Figure 12-1. Prevalence of metabolic syndrome increases with age. (Adapted from Ford ES, Giles WH, Dietz WH: Prevalence of the metabolic syndrome among U.S. adults: Findings from the Third National Health and Nutrition Examination Survey. JAMA 287:356, 2002.)

the development of the metabolic syndrome, even after adjustment for major confounders (age, BMI, smoking, alcohol intake, and socioeconomic status) and potentially mediating factors (insulin, glucose, lipids, and blood pressure).

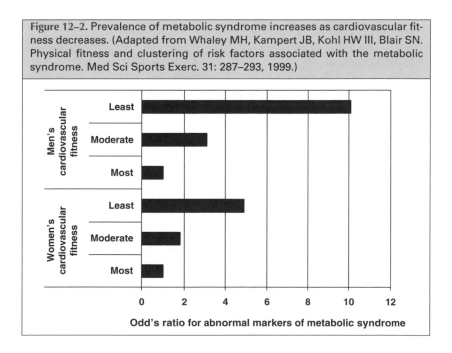

Figure 12-2. Prevalence of metabolic syndrome increases as cardiovascular fitness decreases. (Adapted from Whaley MH, Kampert JB, Kohl HW III, Blair SN. Physical fitness and clustering of risk factors associated with the metabolic syndrome. Med Sci Sports Exerc. 31: 287–293, 1999.)

Common Metabolic Pathways

Epidemiological and clinical research have identified physical inactivity, excessive calorie consumption, and excess weight as common risk factors for both type 2 diabetes and CHD, and have determined that this triad forms the environmental substrate for the metabolic and IR syndromes. Analogous to the concept of a metabolic cluster resulting in these disorders, there exists a cluster of biochemical and metabolic pathways underlying the pathophysiology of inactivity-related disorders. The following two hypotheses, based upon epidemiological data, support this concept:

Hypothesis #1: The phenotypic expression of insulin resistance in sedentary skeletal muscle initiates whole-body insulin resistance, which in turn is associated with atherosclerosis, hypertension, truncal obesity, and type 2 diabetes. Skeletal muscle insulin resistance is likely the manifestation of an inadequately stimulated genotype that is used to seeing a certain dose of an environmental trigger (i.e., physical activity) to maintain normal physiology, and hence prevent pathology. In this sense, physical inactivity is a molecular mechanism of disease in its role as an environmental trigger to modify the evolutionarily programmed genome.

Hypothesis #2: The primary mechanistic hypothesis in the STRRIDE clinical trial[6] is that alterations in skeletal muscle (specifically, skeletal muscle capillarity) mediate most, if not all, of the favorable adaptations in glucose and lipid metabolism mediated by chronic exercise training. STRRIDE's alternative hypothesis is that other stable changes in body habitus induced by exercise training—such as reductions in visceral body fat—account for the majority of the favorable changes in whole body metabolic state, such as insulin action and serum lipids.

For example, our Paleolithically programmed genomes expect a certain threshold of physical activity for their proper expression and function. If inadequate stimulation of the genome occurs secondary to physical inactivity or via excess caloric intake, then there might be a dysregulation of established homeostasis, which ultimately could lead to the metabolic derangement manifested as the metabolic syndrome and/or insulin resistance/hyperinsulinemia (Fig. 12–3).

Physical Inactivity Leads To the Metabolic and Insulin Resistant Syndromes

Insulin sensitivity is directly proportional to maximal aerobic capacity in healthy non-obese subjects.

A significant relationship exists between the level of maximal aerobic ca-

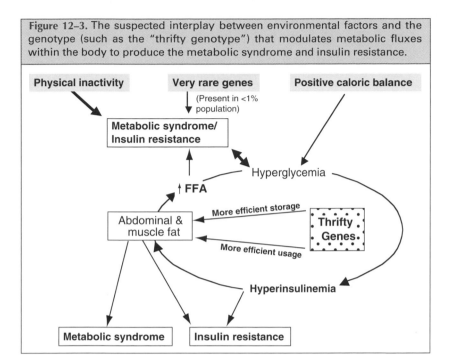

Figure 12-3. The suspected interplay between environmental factors and the genotype (such as the "thrifty genotype") that modulates metabolic fluxes within the body to produce the metabolic syndrome and insulin resistance.

pacity and in vivo insulin-stimulated glucose utilization during an insulin clamp. This effect is independent of age and obesity, and accounts for over 40% of the variance in insulin-stimulated glucose utilization among these subjects. In addition, significant correlations exist between maximal aerobic capacity and the insulin responses to an oral glucose load.[7]

An increase in physical activity improves insulin action in obesity with and without concomitant changes in weight and/or body composition. A review article of random clinical trails concluded that an increase in physical activity by aerobic exercise improved insulin action without weight loss.[8] This is an important point, as it shows that physical activity is as efficacious in disease risk reduction as losing body weight.

Inactivity as a cause of insulin resistance has been overlooked by much of the medical community. The relationship between maximal aerobic capacity and insulin action does not seem well appreciated. Overemphasis on obesity as a cause of insulin resistance has neglected the fact that overweight individuals are often sedentary. Indeed, only ~25% of obese individuals are insulin resistant, and abdominal obesity is not a usual manifestation of the IR syndrome (see Table 12–2). Physical inactivity is a major etiologic factor in the pathogenesis of insulin resistance. Differences in the degree of obesity and the level of maximal aerobic capacity are *both*

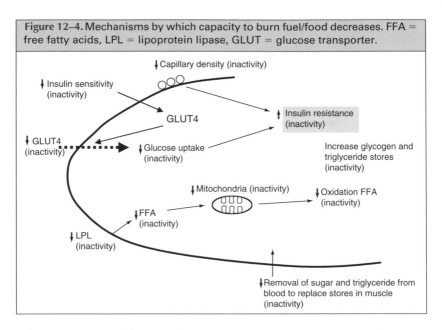

Figure 12–4. Mechanisms by which capacity to burn fuel/food decreases. FFA = free fatty acids, LPL = lipoprotein lipase, GLUT = glucose transporter.

potent in the modulation of insulin-mediated glucose removal in normal subjects.

There is a pathophysiological sequence by which physical inactivity predisposes to a cluster of metabolic diseases.

When our genes do not receive adequate doses of physical activity, skeletal muscle downregulates its capacity to convert blood glucose and fatty acids to ATP. This is analogous to downsizing from a jet engine to a 4-cylinder engine, thereby decreasing the capacity to burn fuel (Fig 12–4).

1. Inactive skeletal muscle's impaired ability to oxidize glucose and fatty acids is mediated by:

- Decreased mitochondrial concentration
- Reduced ability to remove glucose from blood. Decreased glucose removal is the result of fewer capillaries (less glucose can be delivered to the muscle), reduced GLUT4 protein (less glucose can be transferred into the muscle), and reduced insulin stimulation of glucose uptake into the muscle by decreasing insulin signaling to translocate GLUT4 to the cell membrane (termed insulin resistance).
- Reduced ability to hydrolyze blood triglycerides to free fatty acids (secondary to decreased lipoprotein lipase [LPL] activity) that can be taken into the skeletal muscle is also a factor.

2. Inactive skeletal muscle's impaired ability to adequately remove blood glucose and fatty acids consequently results in hyperinsulinemia and hypertriglyceridemia, ultimately leading to increased CHD risk (Fig.

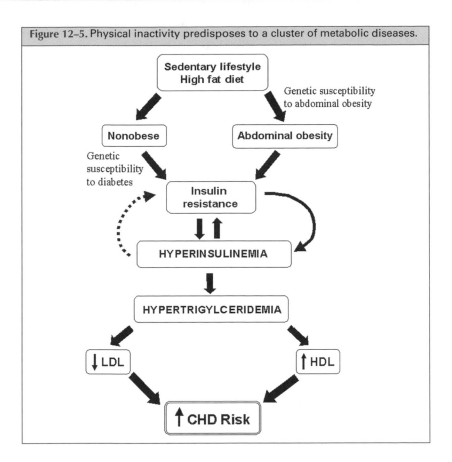

Figure 12–5. Physical inactivity predisposes to a cluster of metabolic diseases.

12–5). β-cells in the pancreas sense the increased blood glucose and release insulin. However, the inactive skeletal muscle has full glycogen stores, and via a yet-to-be-described sequence of events, the inactive muscle becomes resistant to insulin, thereby setting up the spiral of hyperinsulinemia.

Physical activity is a primary and secondary preventive therapy for the metabolic and insulin resistance syndromes.

Physical activity is a potent modality to affect not only the whole cluster of metabolic disorders, but also each one of the components of the metabolic/insulin resistance syndromes.

Suggested Reading

1. Expert Panel on Detection, Evaluation, and Treatment of High Blood Cholesterol in Adults. Executive Summary of the Third Report of the National Cholesterol Education

Program (NCEP) Expert Panel on Detection, Evaluation, and Treatment of High Blood Cholesterol in Adults (Adult Treatment Panel III). JAMA 285:2486, 2002.

2. Reaven G. Metabolic syndrome: Pathophysiology and implications for management of cardiovascular disease. Circulation 106:286–288, 2002.

3. Ford ES, Giles WH, Dietz WH. Prevalence of the metabolic syndrome among U.S. adults: Findings from the Third National Health and Nutrition Examination Survey. JAMA 287:356, 2002.

4. Whaley MH, Kampert JB, Kohl HW III, Blair SN. Physical fitness and clustering of risk factors associated with the metabolic syndrome. Med Sci Sports Exerc. 31: 287–293, 1999.

5. Laaksonen DE, Lakka HM, Salonen JT, et al. Low levels of leisure-time physical activity and cardiorespiratory fitness predict development of the metabolic syndrome. Diabetes Care 25:1612, 2002.

6. Kraus WE, Torgan CE, Duscha BD, et al. Studies of a targeted risk reduction intervention through defined exercise (STRRIDE). Med Sci Sports Exerc 33: 1774–1784, 2001.

7. Rosenthal M, Haskell WL, Solomon R, et al. Demonstration of a relationship between level of physical training and insulin-stimulated glucose utilization in normal humans. Diabetes 32: 408–411, 1983.

8. Kelley DE, Goodpaster BH. Effects of physical activity on insulin action and glucose tolerance in obesity. Med Sci Sports Exerc 31: S619–623, 1999.

Cardiovascular Diseases

Coronary Heart Disease

Epidemiology

Cardiovascular disease (CVD) was the primary cause of 949,619 deaths (41% of all deaths) in the U.S. in 1998, according to the American Heart Association (AHA). Coronary heart disease (CHD) is the number one cause of death in the U.S. today. The Expert Panel on Detection, Evaluation, and Treatment of High Blood Cholesterol in Adults (ATPIII)[1] concluded that: "Physical inactivity is a major, underlying risk factor for coronary artery disease. Physical inactivity augments the lipid and non-lipid risk factors of the metabolic syndrome. Physical inactivity further may enhance risk by impairing cardiovascular fitness and coronary blood flow. Regular physical activity reduces very low-density lipoprotein levels, raises HDL cholesterol, and in some persons, lowers LDL levels. It also can lower blood pressure, reduce insulin resistance, and favorably influence cardiovascular function. Thus, ATP III recommends that regular physical activity become a routine component in management of high serum cholesterol." (See Chapter 14, "Metabolic Diseases," for a detailed discussion of blood lipids.)

According to one study,[2] 35% of all CHD deaths in 1986 were due to the presence of the risk factor of "no regular exercise." Likewise, 29% of all stroke deaths in 1986 occurred to those who had "no regular exercise." Moderate physical activity decreased the prevalence of CHD and stroke by 30% in 72,488 Harvard female nurses,[3,4] compared to no physical activity. In this study, moderate physical activity consisted of > 2.5 hours of brisk walking (> 3 mph) each week.

Physical activity (at least 30 min/day most days of the week) in 30% of the population prevents 68,937 premature deaths and 113,736 cases of CHD and stroke (refer back to Table 4–3). If the 30% reduction in the prevalence of CHD and stroke by undertaking moderate-intensity physical activity were to be extended to the 70% of the population that is sedentary, then 160,852 additional premature deaths and 379,121 cases of CHD and stroke would be prevented annually in the U.S. Additional deaths could be avoided if Americans undertook 1 hour of walking each day, or 30 minutes of jogging/day.

Primary Prevention of Coronary Heart Disease

Patients can be educated about risk factors and helpful lifestyle changes. Programs such as "Choose to Move" by the AHA (see Chapter 11 and http://www.choosetomove.org/about.html) have proven to be useful in this regard. Identify at-risk patients and convince them to alter risky behavior to prevent the development of coronary artery disease (CAD). Most patients with CAD were without CAD at an earlier age. Thus, nearly 100% of the population was eligible for primary prevention when they were infants. Primary prevention must start with the parents of infants and continue through pre-school and nursery school, so that it becomes as automatic as stopping and looking both ways before crossing the street.

We go beyond the recent goal of the AHA, which is that all adults should know the levels and significance of risk factors as assessed by their primary care provider. We think that elementary school children also should know the significance of CAD risk factors. Education is the key!

Here are the American Heart Association guidelines to prevent heart attack and stroke*:
- No exposure to tobacco smoke
- Blood pressure maintained < 140/90 mmHg; < 130/85 mmHg for people with kidney damage or heart failure; < 130/80 mmHg for people with diabetes
- An overall healthy eating pattern
- Cholesterol lowered to appropriate level based upon individual risk (LDL-C < 100 mg/dl for established CHD and diabetes)
- *At least 30 minutes of moderate-intensity physical activity on most (preferably all) days of the week*
- Achieve and maintain desirable BMI of 18.5–24.9 kg/m^2
- Normal fasting blood glucose (< 110 mg/mL).
- Regular pulse checks and treatment for atrial fibrillation, an irregular heartbeat associated with blood clot formation, which could lead to stroke.

Secondary Prevention of CHD

Unfortunately, much of the U.S. population requires secondary preventive efforts. Approximately 60% of overweight (body mass index

---

*http://www.americanheart.org/presenter.jhtml?identifier=4704

[BMI] > 95th percentile) youth, including children aged 5 to 10 years, have at least one risk factor for future CVD, including blood pressure elevation, abnormal lipids, and insulin elevation, and more than 25% have two or more of these risk factors. Thus, all overweight children/adolescents must have secondary preventive reductions in CVD risk. The parents of these children should be counseled to reduce time in sedentary activities such as TV viewing, and parents should engage children in more play. (See Chapter 5 for details on prevention in children.)

The American Heart Association has just released the recommendation that screening for heart disease be started at the age of 20 years. They advise determining the need for secondary prevention by:

- Updating family history of CHD regularly
- Assessing smoking status, diet, alcohol intake, and physical activity at every routine evaluation
- Recording blood pressure, BMI, waist circumference, and pulse (to screen for atrial fibrillation) at each visit (at least every 2 years)
- Measuring fasting serum lipoprotein profile and fasting blood glucose at least every 5 years; if risk factors are present, every 2 years.

The AHA has issued these recommendations for patients older than 40:

- These patients should know their absolute risk of developing CHD.
- Adults, especially those with two or more risk factors, should have their 10-year risk of CHD assessed with a multiple risk factor score every 5 years (or more often if risk factors change)
- Risk factors used in the global risk assessment should include: age, gender, smoking status, *physical activity level,* systolic (sometimes diastolic) blood pressure, total (and sometimes LDL) cholesterol, HDL cholesterol, and, in some risk scores, diabetes. (Note: we include physical inactivity here because the AHA included it elsewhere in their recommendations.)
- A patient with established diabetes, or a 10-year risk for diabetes over 20%, can be considered "CHD equivalent," which is to say that he or she has a risk profile similar to a patient with established CHD.

Tertiary Prevention of CHD

Remarkably, in a study by Hambrecht et al,[5] 4 weeks of exercise training by 60-year-old patients with CHD attenuated the paradoxical vasoconstriction in response to acetylcholine in epicardial coronary vessels and resistance vessels. This occurred by an increase in endothelium-dependent vasodilatation (Fig. 13–1), which led to a 500% increase in coronary blood flow (Fig. 13–2). The exercise training was six times/wk for 10 min at 80% of $\dot{V}O_2$ max, with 10 minutes total of warm-up and cooldown.

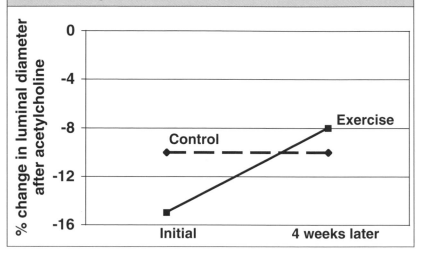

Figure 13–1. The effect of exercise on endothelium-dependent vasodilatation in 60-year-old patients. (Adapted from Hambrecht R, Wolf A, Gielen S, et al: Effect of exercise on coronary endothelial function in patients with coronary artery disease. New Engl J Med 342:454–460, 2000.)

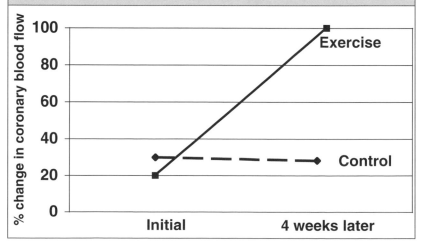

Figure 13–2. The effect of exercise on coronary blood flow in 60-year-old patients. (Adapted from Hambrecht R, Wolf A, Gielen S, et al: Effect of exercise on coronary endothelial function in patients with coronary artery disease. New Engl J Med 342:454–460, 2000.)

Acceleration of Atherosclerosis

Physical inactivity accelerates the development of atherosclerosis by producing endothelial dysfunction (Fig. 13–3). Vascular endothelial cells form a one-cell-thick layer that lines all of our blood vessels. Endothelial production of nitric oxide (NO) exerts vasoprotective effects on the vascular wall (Table 13–1). The endothelium is highly regulated, and hence can be modulated by a variety of factors (Table 13–2).[6]

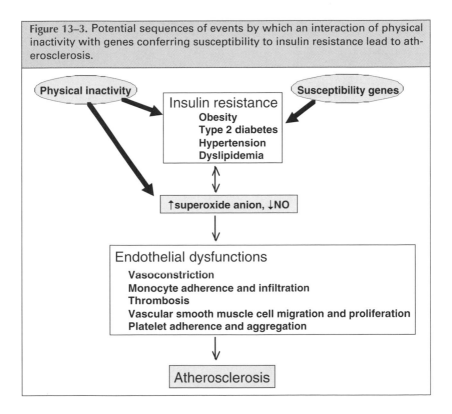

Figure 13–3. Potential sequences of events by which an interaction of physical inactivity with genes conferring susceptibility to insulin resistance lead to atherosclerosis.

Category	Healthy Endothelium	Endothelial Dysfunction
TABLE 13–1. Healthy Endothelium Vs. Endothelial Dysfunction		
Blood vessel size	Vasodilation	Vasoconstriction
Monocyte adherence and infiltration of capillary wall	Prevents	Potentiates
Platelet adhesion and aggregration	Prevents	Potentiates
Clotting (thrombosis)	Fibrinolysis	Coagulation
Smooth muscle cell proliferation and migration	Prevents	Potentiates
Oxidative stress	Prevents	Potentiates

TABLE 13–2. Factors Altering Endothelial Health

Promotes Endothelial Health	Potentiates Endothelial Dysfunction
Physical activity	Physical inactivity
ACE inhibitors	Tobacco
Calcium channel blockers	Hypertension
Statins	Hypercholesterolemia
NO donors and arginine	Diabetes mellitus
Antioxidants	Aging
Aspirin	Asymmetric dimethyl arginine
Estrogens	Homocysteinemia

Adapted from Wroblewski Lissin L, Cooke JP: Maintaining the endothelium: Preventive strategies for vessel integrity. Prev Cardiol 3:172–177, 2000.

Physical activity-mediated health outcome and physical inactivity–mediated disease effect on endothelial cells is transmitted via NO, and possibly also through prostaglandin PGI_2 and endothelium-derived hyperpolarizing factor. NO increases with physical activity and decreases with physical inactivity. In fact, a *single day* of increased physical activity increases NO, with a resultant beneficial effect on endothelial health (see Table 13–3; though very similar to Table 13–1, it highlights the effects of physical activity).

Pathways By Which Increased Physical Activity Improves Endothelial Health

A variety of diseases are associated with an impairment of endothelium-dependent NO activity. One of the major causes is believed to be an increased production of reactive oxygen species, in particular superoxide, which have been shown to interfere with many steps of the NO-cyclic guanosine monophosphate (cGMP) pathway. Increased production of reactive oxygen species has been found in diverse conditions such as

TABLE 13–3. Effects On Endothelial Health By Changes in Quantity of Nitric Oxide

Category	Increased Endothelial NO Due To Physical Activity	Decreased Endothelial NO Due To Physical *In*activity
Blood vessel size	Vasodilation	Vasoconstriction
Monocyte adherence and infiltration of capillary wall	Prevents	Potentiates
Platelet adhesion and aggregration	Prevents	Potentiates
Coagulation	Prevents	Potentiates
Smooth muscle cell proliferation and migration	Prevents	Potentiates
Oxidative stress	Prevents	Potentiates

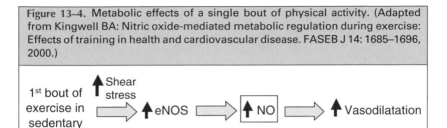

Figure 13–4. Metabolic effects of a single bout of physical activity. (Adapted from Kingwell BA: Nitric oxide-mediated metabolic regulation during exercise: Effects of training in health and cardiovascular disease. FASEB J 14: 1685–1696, 2000.)

atherosclerosis, hypertension, diabetes, hypercholesterolemia, heart failure, cigarette smoking, and physical inactivity.

A single bout of physical activity increases shear stress from the increased coronary blood flow experienced by endothelial cells, which subsequently results in increased NO production via endothelial nitric oxide synthase (eNOS) stimulation, ultimately causing coronary vasodilatation (Fig. 13–4).[7] Conversely, physical *in*activity produces vascular endothelial dysfunction by acutely *decreasing* NO production from existing eNOS and, more chronically, by reducing eNOS (Fig. 13–5). Note that repeated daily physical activity further improves and, more importantly, *maintains* the health of coronary blood vessels (Fig. 13–6).

Remember that the biochemical processes underlying this dramatic effect of physical activity on coronary vessel health are due to acetylcholine-mediated release of NO, which in turn diffuses to adjacent smooth muscle

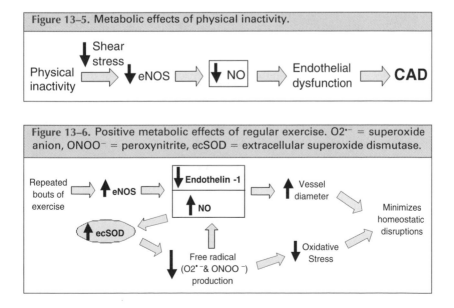

Figure 13–5. Metabolic effects of physical inactivity.

Figure 13–6. Positive metabolic effects of regular exercise. $O2^{\bullet-}$ = superoxide anion, $ONOO^{-}$ = peroxynitrite, ecSOD = extracellular superoxide dismutase.

cells and relaxes them (vasodilation). Most heart diseases are associated with dysfunctional endothelial cells that cannot produce enough NO to relax the smooth muscle surrounding blood vessels, and thus vasoconstriction occurs. Physical activity rescues the endothelium from dysfunction by increasing both eNOS and extracellular superoxide dismutase (ecSOD) expression, thereby producing more NO, which in turn increases myocardial perfusion in patients with stable coronary artery disease (Fig. 13–7). Upregulation of eNOS and ecSOD occurs only after *repeated* daily increases in physical activity, not in a single active episode.

The increases in ecSOD and other antioxidant enzymes by repeated daily bouts of physical activity protect NO from degradation, thereby accentuating coronary vessel vasodilation. For example, 3 weeks of treadmill training increased eNOS protein expression in mouse aortas by about three-fold, with a similar concomitant increase in the expression of ecSOD protein, compared to sedentary mice.[8] In striking contrast to these results in wild-type mice, exercise training had no effect on ecSOD protein levels in mice completely lacking the eNOS gene,[8] implying that NO signaled increased ecSOD expression. The consequences of the upregulation of ecSOD in response to NO in normal mice would be to reduce reactions of NO with superoxide anion, thereby extending the lifespan of NO and enhancing its biologic effects. In addition, upregulation of ecSOD expression by NO very likely represents an important feed-forward mechanism, whereby NO released from the endothelium ultimately enhanced its own biologic effect by reducing superoxide anion.

The enhanced endothelium-dependent vasodilator reserve that develops with exercise training over months is most likely related to blood lipid profile modification. Hypercholesterolemia, free fatty acids, and

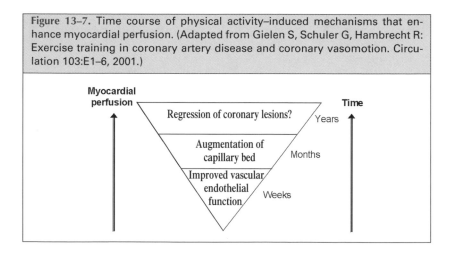

Figure 13–7. Time course of physical activity–induced mechanisms that enhance myocardial perfusion. (Adapted from Gielen S, Schuler G, Hambrecht R: Exercise training in coronary artery disease and coronary vasomotion. Circulation 103:E1–6, 2001.)

oxidized lipids all produce endothelial dysfunction, which ultimately leads to coronary and peripheral vascular disease. *Increased physical activity increases blood HDL and lowers triglycerides.* In contrast, physical *in*activity is associated with lowered expression of both eNOS and ecSOD proteins, less vasodilation, higher oxidative stress, and more endothelial dysfunction in coronary blood vessels.

Other Cardiovascular Consequences of Physical Activity

Reduces arterial stiffness. Large-artery compliance is increased (decreased stiffness) immediately after an acute exercise bout.[22] Moreover, 4 weeks of moderate aerobic exercise has been shown to increase large-artery compliance in young normotensive, but previously sedentary subjects. On the other hand, sedentary individuals have a reduced large-artery compliance, i.e., stiffer vessels, than do endurance-trained counterparts. Aerobic fitness, total cholesterol, and LDL-cholesterol were all found to be significant *independent* physiological correlates of central arterial stiffness in healthy females varying in age and physical activity status.[23]

Reduces ischemia and injury. Physical activity also appears to exert an acute protective effect in heart muscle. A single 30-minute bout of running by rats on a treadmill conferred a cardioprotective effect on the myocardium that resulted in a limitation of infarct size 24 hours later.[24] Pharmacological inhibition of protein kinase C activation during the exercise period abrogated this protective response. Exercise has also been shown to reduce ischemia/reperfusion injury to the heart of rats by up-regulating tumor necrosis factor (TNF-β), interleukin 1 (IL-1β), and manganese-superoxide dismutase (Mn-SOD), all of which are known to be cardioprotectants. Mn-SOD is an intrinsic radical scavenger, while TNF and IL-1 are inducers of Mn-SOD.[25]

Reduces atherosclerosis. Physically active primates have a lower incidence of atherosclerosis.[9] Although serum total cholesterol was the same (~ 600 mg/dl) in exercising and non-exercising monkeys on an atherogenic diet, the physically active monkeys, even on this diet, had significantly higher HDL cholesterol and much lower triglyceride and LDL plus VLDL triglyceride levels. Ischemic electrocardiographic changes, angiographic signs of coronary artery narrowing, and sudden death were observed only in physically *in*active monkeys, in which post-mortem examination revealed marked coronary atherosclerosis and stenoses. Physical activity was associated with substantially reduced overall atherosclerotic involvement, lesion size, and collagen accumulation. The physically active monkeys also had much larger hearts and wider coronary arteries, further reducing the degree of luminal narrowing. *Thus, moderate-intensity physical activity significantly prevents or retards CHD in primates.*

Physical Activity Reduces Inflammatory Mediators

Inflammatory mediators that are thought to be involved in the development and progression of CHD are reduced by physical activity. Recent data from the Women's Health Initiative prospective study of 75,343 women[20] demonstrated that C-reactive protein (CRP) and IL-6 are *independent predictors* of CAD among these apparently healthy postmenopausal women. While hormone replacement therapy (HRT) is known to increase CRP, one of the striking findings of this study was that use or nonuse of HRT had *less* importance as a predictor of cardiovascular risk than did baseline levels of either CRP or IL-6. Thus, even after adjusting for total cholesterol/HDL and all other risk factors, the odds ratio for CAD significantly increased with increasing CRP levels.

Remarkably, physical activity can decrease CRP, along with many of the other inflammatory mediators. In a representative sample of 16,000 U.S. adults,[21] progressive increases in leisure-time physical activity resulted in decreased blood CRP, fibrinogen concentration, and white blood cell (WBC) count, but with increased albumin concentration. This physical activity–induced decrease in CRP levels suggests that physical activity may reduce inflammation. Inflammation is considered to be critical in the pathogenesis of atherosclerotic disease (Fig. 13–8).

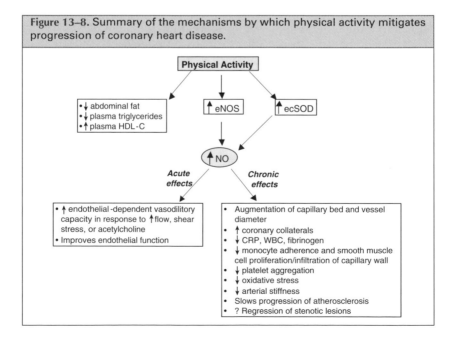

Figure 13–8. Summary of the mechanisms by which physical activity mitigates progression of coronary heart disease.

Congestive Heart Failure

Epidemiology

The incidence of congestive heart failure (CHF) has been steadily increasing over the last 10 years. Today, 4.6 million individuals in the U.S. have CHF; 400,000 new cases are added annually; and 43,000 individuals die of CHF.[11] Hospitalizations for CHF increased from 377,000 to 870,000 between the years 1979 and 1996.[11] CHF is a multifactorial condition, and some of its precipitating causes are: coronary artery disease (60%), hypertension (10%), physical inactivity (9%), obesity (8%), and diabetes (3%). Lack of physical activity is considered an independent risk factor for the development of CHF. In fact, bed rest and exercise restriction lead to deconditioning and increased morbidity in patients with symptomatic heart failure. Therefore, physical inactivity can exacerbate conditions associated with previously diagnosed CHF.

Tertiary Prevention

Patients diagnosed with CHF benefit greatly from participating in exercise training programs. For example, exercise training of patients with moderate to severe CHF lowered all-cause mortality by 63% and reduced hospital readmission for heart failure by 71%![12] While the primary defective organ in CHF is the heart, the peripheral musculature becomes a secondary defective organ of major clinical significance, in that skeletal muscle, rather than the congestive heart, appears to limit exercise tolerance. In the heart failure syndrome, two of the main symptoms are *fatigue* and *limitation in exercise capacity*. In many heart failure patients, an inherent defect in skeletal muscle function is operative, rather than a hemodynamic limitation (Fig. 13–9).[13]

The evidence is quite clear that exercise training improves the overall function and exercise capacity of people inflicted with CHF.[26] Exercise capacity correlates well with measures of peripheral muscular strength

Figure 13–9. Effect of physical inactivity on skeletal muscle in CHF. ECC= excitation-contraction coupling in skeletal muscle. (Adapted from Tavazzi L, Giannuzzi P. Physical training as a therapeutic measure in chronic heart failure: Time for recommendations. Heart 86: 7–11, 2001.)

CHF patients without physical activity		Changes in expression of various ECC proteins		↑Skeletal muscle fatigue (hallmark feature in CHF)

and endurance (r = 0.90), which suggests that alterations in the periphery greatly contribute to exercise intolerance in CHF patients. Exercise training does *not* improve function of the primary defective organ, i.e., the heart. Only moderate improvements are noted in left ventricular performance or central hemodynamics after exercise training in CHF patients. Therefore, reductions in exercise capacity observed in CHF patients are *not* due solely to alterations in myocardial function. For example, various indicators of cardiac function (e.g., ejection fraction) do not correlate well (r = −0.06) with overall exercise capacity. The fact remains, however, these same patients do exhibit significant improvements in overall exercise capacity, as skeletal muscle dysfunction in CHF does improve with exercise training. Physically active skeletal muscles generally mean improved quality of life for these patients. Exercise training often improves their condition, while physical *in*activity may actually increase their risk of mortality.

Biochemical Mechanisms

We have just described the physiological mechanisms by which physical inactivity affects patients with CHF. Now let us turn our attention to how physical activity can improve function in this disease. Simply put, increased blood flow improves mitochondrial function, which raises functional capacity and reduces skeletal muscle fatigue (Fig. 13–10).

As for biochemical mechanisms: Oxidative stress in the congestive heart produces endothelial dysfunction. Usage of an endothelial cell inhibitor of xanthine oxidase, allopurinol, in CHF patients improved

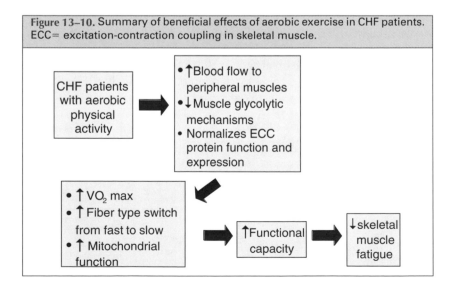

Figure 13–10. Summary of beneficial effects of aerobic exercise in CHF patients. ECC= excitation-contraction coupling in skeletal muscle.

CHF patients with aerobic physical activity →
- ↑Blood flow to peripheral muscles
- ↓Muscle glycolytic mechanisms
- Normalizes ECC protein function and expression

- ↑ VO_2 max
- ↑ Fiber type switch from fast to slow
- ↑ Mitochondrial function

→ ↑Functional capacity → ↓skeletal muscle fatigue

endothelium-dependent vasodilation and exercise capacity.[14] The congestive failing heart produces NO from inducible NOS, whose blockage enhances myocardial contractility, but inhibition of NOS does not affect contractility in the normal heart.[15]

Hypertension

Epidemiology

From a meta-analysis of 44 randomized trials of physical training, it was concluded that physically inactive populations had blood pressures that were higher by 2/3 (systolic/diastolic) mmHg in normotensive subjects and by 7/6 mmHg in hypertensive patients as compared to the physically active groups.[16]

Intermediate Mechanisms

Thirty minutes of brisk walking 5 to 7 times per week for 12 weeks by mild, untreated essential-hypertension patients lowered their systolic and diastolic blood pressures and increased forearm blood flow in response to the infusion of acetylcholine[27] (see Coronary Heart Disease section in this chapter for discussion of acetylcholine-induced vasodilation and endothelial dysfunction). This response was blocked by a NO inhibitor, suggesting a role for NO. Less NO would favor vasoconstriction. Plasma nitrate (an index of NO quantity) was lower in sedentary hypertensive rats compared to those allowed access to 35 days of voluntary wheel running.[28]

There was an inverse relationship between the decrease in ratio of total cholesterol to HDL cholesterol and the increase in maximal forearm blood flow response to acetylcholine after the 12-wk training in hypertensive patients, suggesting that high cholesterol causes endothelial dysfunction.[27]

Resting levels of circulating norepinephrine were higher in sedentary subjects than physically active subjects.[27] Norepinephrine produces peripheral vasoconstriction and increases total peripheral resistance. Sedentary hypertensive rats had increased adrenergic agent–induced vasoconstrictor responses that were associated with an attenuated NO release in thoracic aortas and carotid arteries relative to exercise-trained hypertensive rats.[29]

Currently, little information describing cellular mechanisms is available.

Stroke

Epidemiology

Physical inactivity increases the risk of ischemic stroke.[30] A higher risk of cerebrovascular accidents is present in the sedentary elderly than in the elderly who are physically active.[31] A Statement for Healthcare Professionals From the Stroke Council of the American Heart Association made the recommendation that, as per guidelines endorsed by the CDC and the NIH, regular exercise (> 30 minutes of moderate-intensity activity daily) is part of a healthy lifestyle and helps to reduce comorbid conditions that may lead to stroke.[30] Note that the effect of physical activity's prevention of stroke seems more convincing for ischemic stroke than for hemorrhagic stroke.

Biochemical/Cellular Mechanisms

It has been suggested that the protective effect of physical activity may be partly mediated through its effects on various risk factors for stroke. Physical activity lowers blood pressure, facilitates weight loss and

Figure 13–11. Potential sequence of events showing how physical activity may lead to a decreased risk of stroke.

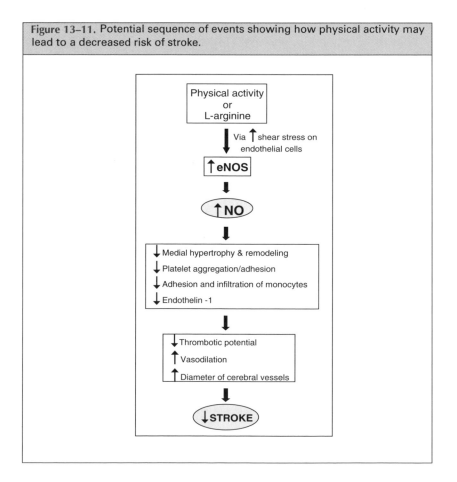

weight maintenance, increases serum HDL cholesterol, is associated with reductions in plasma fibrinogen level and platelet aggregation, and elevates plasma tissue plasminogen activator activity (Fig. 13–11).

Physical inactivity precipitates abnormal endothelial cell function, much in the same way as described for CAD. Endothelial dysfunction is due to a selective abnormality of NO synthesis, probably related to a defect in the phosphatidylinositol/Ca^{2+} signaling pathway. NO, a potent vasodilator, is produced by the endothelium of cerebral arteriolar resistance vessels and is crucial to maintaining appropriate cerebral perfusion.

Intermittent Claudication

Epidemiology

The age-adjusted prevalence of peripheral arterial disease is approximately 12% for those older than 60. A meta-analysis of 21 studies found that the average time or walking distance to the onset and peak of claudication pain increased 179% and 122%, respectively, following a program of exercise rehabilitation.[17] Exercise improves functional status while undertaking activities of daily living.

Biochemical/Cellular Mechanisms

Exercise training is not associated with substantial changes in blood flow to the legs, and the changes that do occur poorly predict the clinical response. However, exercise training improves oxygen extraction in the legs independent of alterations in blood flow, likely through improvements in intermediary metabolism of skeletal muscle. It also improves gait and walking efficiency, which then lowers the O_2 cost for a given workload.

NOS inhibition has been shown to block arteriogenesis in response to exercise, but not angiogenesis, in peripheral arterial insufficiency.

One hour of acute, submaximal treadmill running resulted in a fourfold increase in vascular endotheial growth factor mRNA in an *NO-dependent manner,* and more modest increases in transforming growth factor-1 and basic fibroblast growth factor mRNA in the rat gastrocnemius muscle.[18]

Platelet Adhesion and Aggregation

Epidemiology

Sedentary individuals have higher platelet adhesion and aggregation at rest or during the first bout of exercise, compared to a group undertaking regular low- to moderate-intensity physical activity on a daily basis.[19] These effects are activity-dependent, as deconditioning for 30 days largely reversed these training effects back to the pretraining state.

Biochemical Mechanisms

Wang et al[19] showed that exercise training in women at the midfollicular phase of their menstrual cycle enhanced plasma nitrite and nitrate and platelet cGMP levels, while at the same time suppressing basal and ADP-induced platelet $[Ca^{2+}]$ elevation. Together, these events have been shown to suppress platelet reactivity. Currently, little information is available describing other cellular mechanisms.

Suggested Reading

1. Executive Summary of The Third Report of The National Cholesterol Education Program (NCEP) Expert Panel on Detection, Evaluation, And Treatment of High Blood Cholesterol In Adults (Adult Treatment Panel III). JAMA 285:2486–2497, 2001.
2. Hahn RA, Teutsch SM, Rothenberg RB, Marks JS. Excess deaths from nine chronic diseases in the United States, 1986. JAMA 264:2654–2659, 1990.
3. Manson JE, Hu FB, Rich-Edwards JW, et al. A prospective study of walking as compared with vigorous exercise in the prevention of coronary heart disease in women. N Engl J Med 341: 650–658, 1999.
4. Hu FB, Stampfer MJ, Colditz GA, et al. Physical activity and risk of stroke in women. JAMA 283: 2961–2967, 2000.
5. Hambrecht R, Wolf A, Gielen S, et al. Effect of exercise on coronary endothelial function in patients with coronary artery disease. New Engl J Med 342:454–460, 2000.
6. Wroblewski Lissin L, Cooke JP. Maintaining the endothelium: Preventive strategies for vessel integrity. Prev Cardiol 3:172–177, 2000.
7. Kingwell BA. Nitric oxide-mediated metabolic regulation during exercise: Effects of training in health and cardiovascular disease. FASEB J 14: 1685–1696, 2000.
8. Fukai T, Siegfried MR, Ushio-Fukai M, et al. Regulation of the vascular extracellular superoxide dismutase by nitric oxide and exercise training. J Clin Invest 105: 1631–1639, 2000.
9. Kramsch DM, Aspen AJ, Abramowitz BM, et al. Reduction of coronary atherosclerosis by moderate conditioning exercise in monkeys on an atherogenic diet. N Engl J Med. 1981; 305(25):1483–1489.
10. Gielen S, Schuler G, Hambrecht R. Exercise training in coronary artery disease and coronary vasomotion. Circulation 103:E1–6, 2001.
11. American Heart Association: 1999 Heart and Stroke Statistical Update. Dallas, Texas, American Heart Association, 2000.
12. Belardinelli R, Georgiou D, Cianci G, Purcaro A. Randomized, controlled trial of long-term moderate exercise training in chronic heart failure: Effects on functional capacity, quality of life, and clinical outcomes. Circulation 99: 1173–1182, 1999.
13. Tavazzi L, Giannuzzi P. Physical training as a therapeutic measure in chronic heart failure: Time for recommendations. Heart 86: 7–11, 2001.
14. Farquharson CA, Butler R, Hill A, et al. Allopurinol improves endothelial dysfunction in chronic heart failure. Circulation 106:221–226, 2002.

15. Chen Y, Traverse JH, Du R, Hou M, Bache RJ. Nitric oxide modulates myocardial oxygen consumption in the failing heart. Circulation 106:273–279, 2002.
16. Fagard RH. Physical activity in the prevention and treatment of hypertension in the obese. Med Sci Sports Exerc 31: S624–S630, 1999.
17. Gardner AW, Poehlman ET. Exercise rehabilitation programs for the treatment of claudication pain. JAMA 274: 975–980, 1995.
18. Breen EC, Johnson EC, Wagner H, et al. Angiogenic growth factor mRNA responses in muscle to a single bout of exercise. J Appl Physiol 81: 355–361, 1996.
19. Wang JS, Jen CJ, Chen HI. Effects of chronic exercise and deconditioning on platelet function in women. J Appl Physiol 83: 2080–2085, 1997.
20. Pradhan AD, Manson JE, Rossouw JE, et al. Inflammatory Biomarkers, Hormone Replacement Therapy, and Incident Coronary Heart Disease: Prospective Analysis From the Women's Health Initiative Observational Study. JAMA 288:980–987, 2002.
21. Ford ES. Does exercise reduce inflammation? Physical activity and C-reactive protein among U.S. adults. Epidemiology 13:561–568, 2002.
22. Kingwell BA. Large artery stiffness: Implications for exercise capacity and cardiovascular risk. Clin Exp Pharmacol Physiol 29:214–217, 2002.
23. Tanaka H, DeSouza CA, Seals DR. Absence of age-related increase in central arterial stiffness in physically active women. Arterioscler Throm Vasc Biol 18:127–132, 1998.
24. Yamashita N, Baxter GF, Yellon. Exercise directly enhances myocardial tolerance to ischaemia-reperfusion injury in the rat through a protein kinase C mediated mechanism. Heart 85:331–336, 2001.
25. Yamashita N, Hoshida S, Otsuk K, et al. Exercise provides direct biphasic cardioprotection via manganese superoxide dismutase activation. J Exp Med 189:1699–1706, 1999.
26. Gielen S, Erbs S, Schuler G, Hambrecht R. Exercise training and endothelial dysfunction in coronary artery disease and chronic heart failure. From molecular biology to clinical benefits. Minerva Cardioangiol 50:95–106, 2002.
27. Higashi Y, Sasaki S, Kurisu S, et al. Regular aerobic exercise augments endothelium-dependent vascular relaxation in normotensive as well as hypertensive subjects: Role of endothelium-derived nitric oxide. Circulation 100:1194–1202, 1999.
28. Jonsdottir IH, Jungersten L, Johansson C, et al. Increase in nitric oxide formation after chronic voluntary exercise in spontaneously hypertensive rats. Acta Physiol Scand 162:149–153, 1998.
29. Chen HI, Chiang IP. Chronic exercise decreases agonist-induced vasoconstriction in spontaneously hypertensive rats. Am J Physiol 271:H977–H983, 1996.
30. Ingall TJ. Preventing ischemic stroke. Current approaches to primary and secondary prevention. Postgrad Med 107:34–50, 2000.
31. Lee CD, Blair SN. Cardiorespiratory fitness and stroke mortality in men. Med Sci Sports Exerc 34:592–595, 2002.

Metabolic Diseases

chapter
14

Type 2 Diabetes

Epidemiology

The prevalence of type 2 diabetes continues to increase among U.S. adults, and the disorder is classified as an "epidemic" by the Centers for Disease Control and Prevention (CDC).[1] The CDC estimates that if undiagnosed cases are included, 10% of the U.S. adult population has type 2 diabetes. In 1958, approximately 1.3 million individuals had type 2 diabetes; in 1998, the number was closer to 10 million (Fig. 14–1). Some of

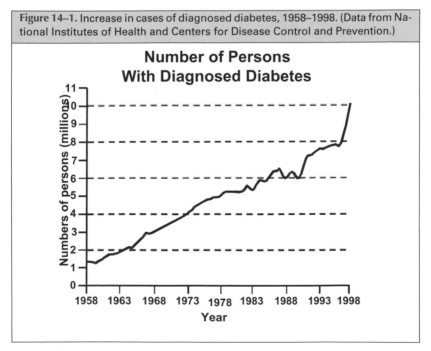

Figure 14–1. Increase in cases of diagnosed diabetes, 1958–1998. (Data from National Institutes of Health and Centers for Disease Control and Prevention.)

Number of Persons With Diagnosed Diabetes

this increase is due to population growth (~57%), but it is unlikely to be due to better diagnostic modalities since neither the techniques nor skills have drastically changed. It also is *not* a result of changed gene structure or mutations, as the human genome has not changed in 10,000 years. In fact, the increase in type 2 diabetes is due to a change in environmental factors (e.g., sedentary lifestyle and nutrition). However, we believe that diet is overemphasized by some who claim it is the sole cause of the epidemic increase in type 2 diabetes.

If a person is physically active, skeletal muscles will remove excessive blood glucose and fats. For example, lumberjacks eat 4500–8000 kcal/day but have a BMI of 25.5 kg/m^2. Lumberjacks are not obese because they expend 4500–8000 kcal/day in physical labor. Compared to the intake of lumberjacks and hunter-gatherers, sedentary individuals "undereat"—but they also "underexercise." Their calorie intake exceeds calorie expenditure, but the current media dogma that sedentary individuals are obese because they overeat is incorrect.

Here is proof that environmental factors (particularly physical inactivity) are the cause of increased type 2 diabetes worldwide:
- Weight loss is not necessary to benefit from the effects of physical activity on glucose tolerance and insulin clearance rates.
- While the overall prevalence of type 2 diabetes in industrialized countries is 6–10%, it is only 0–2% in native populations that have maintained an active lifestyle similar to hunter-gatherer cultures.
- Hu et al[2] found that 91% of the cases of type 2 diabetes in the Harvard Nurse's study could be attributed to habits and forms of behavior that did *not* conform to the low-risk pattern of no smoking; BMI < 25 kg/m^2; consumption of 5–10 g of alcohol per day; moderate-to-vigorous physical activity for at least 30 min/ day; and a score in the highest 40% of the cohort for consumption of a diet high in cereal fiber, marine n-3 fatty acids, and folate, with a high ratio of polyunsaturated to saturated fat and low in trans fat and glycemic load.
- Women with normal body weight and having < 2 MET-hr/wk of total physical activity had twice the risk of type 2 diabetes, as compared to normal-weight women who had > 22 MET-hr/wk of physical activity. Thus, physical inactivity elevates the risk of type 2 diabetes in normal-weight individuals, which reinforces the concept that physical inactivity is an independent risk factor for type 2 diabetes.
- Physically inactive individuals are likely to have a higher BMI, and the prevalence of type 2 diabetes increases with higher BMIs (> 25 kg/m^2).

Type 2 diabetes is preventable. Yet each year there are 798,000 newly diagnosed cases of diabetes and 198,140 deaths attributed to diabetes.

We estimate that 78,923 cases of diabetes and 19,596 deaths are prevented each year in the 30% of the population that are more physically active than the Surgeon General's 30 minutes of moderate activity each day. If the 70% of individuals who now perform < 30 minutes of daily moderate physical activity were to engage in an activity equivalent to brisk walking for at least 30 minutes each day, we estimate that an additional 184,154 cases of diabetes and 45,725 deaths would be prevented each year in this population. Thus, 30 minutes of brisk walking each day by all Americans would lead to 263,077 fewer cases of diabetes and 65,321 fewer deaths. Higher levels of physical activity such as jogging 30 min/day would further reduce the incidence of type 2 diabetes. No current pharmacological approach prevents and reduces the prevalence of type 2 diabetes as effectively as does physical activity.

Primary Prevention of Type 2 Diabetes Mellitus

The CDC asserts that type 2 diabetes is largely preventable by changes in lifestyle. The director of the CDC wrote: "Restoring physical activity to our daily routines is crucial to the future reduction of diabetes and obesity in the U.S. population."[1] The adverse effects of eliminating physical activity and increasing sedentary time (such as TV viewing) are dra-

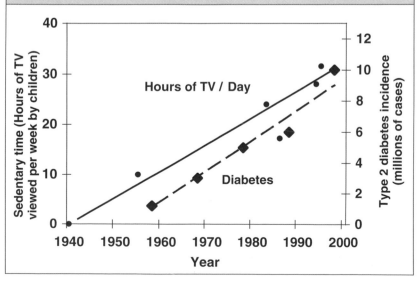

Figure 14–2. In children, the increase in type 2 diabetes (*dashed line*) from 1958 to 1998 correlates with an increase in hours of TV viewed per day (*solid line*) from 1940 to 1995. (Data from Certain LK, Kahn RS: Prevalence, correlates, and trajectory of television viewing among infants and toddlers. Pediatrics 109(4):634–642, 2002.)

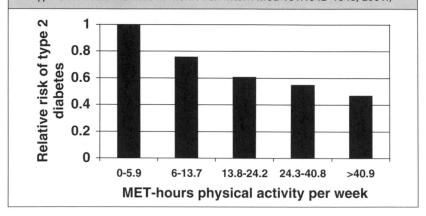

Figure 14–3. In adults, the relative risk of type 2 diabetes was dramatically reduced by increased physical activity. (Adapted from Hu FB, Leitzmann MF, Stampfer MJ, et al: Physical activity and television watching in relation to risk for type 2 diabetes mellitus in men. Arch Intern Med 161:1542–1548, 2001.)

matic. Certain and Kahn's study[3] of TV viewing in childhood (Fig. 14–2) suggests that:

- it initiates biological and behavioral events that facilitate the long pre-clinical period before overt clinical symptoms of type 2 diabetes appear
- it substitutes sedentary time for physically active time.

Hu et al[4] examined the relationship between TV viewing and diabetes in adults: 37,918 health professionals (physicians, dentists, optometrists, pharmacists, podiatrists, osteopaths, and veterinarians) aged 40–75 yrs reported their TV viewing for 10 years, and the data was normalized to 1.0 for the lowest level of weekly physical activity (0–5.9 MET hr/week). The relative risk of type 2 diabetes was dramatically reduced by half in those with > 40.9 MET hr/wk, compared to those engaging in the least physical activity (Fig. 14–3) and most TV viewing time. Every additional

TABLE 14–1. Metabolic Equivalents of Brisk Walking*		
MET Hr/Week	Hours Walking 3 Mph/Week	Minutes Walking 3 Mph/Day
6	2	17
12	4	34
18	6	51
24	8	68
36	12	102

*These values are for a 60-kg individual. An individual weighing 120-kg would only have to walk half as many minutes per day to burn the same number of calories as the 60-kg individual. Walking slower would require longer walks to burn the same number of calories. Walking faster would require less time.

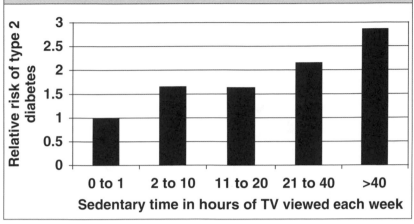

Figure 14–4. Risk of type 2 diabetes rises with increased sedentary time. (Adapted from Hu FB, Leitzmann MF, Stampfer MJ, et al: Physical activity and television watching in relation to risk for type 2 diabetes mellitus in men. Arch Intern Med 161:1542–1548, 2001.)

18 MET hr/wk of physical activity was associated with a 19% reduction in risk of type 2 diabetes. Every 2-hour increment spent watching TV was associated with an additional 50% increase in the risk of diabetes (Fig. 14–4). Those viewing TV the most were at more than twice the risk.

Secondary Prevention of Type 2 Diabetes Mellitus

A large, randomized clinical trial in the U.S.[5] involving 3234 pre-diabetic individuals (i.e., had elevated fasting and postprandial plasma glucose concentrations) showed that the incidence of diabetes was 58% lower in the lifestyle-intervention group and 31% lower in the metformin group, compared to the placebo group. The goals of the lifestyle-modification program were at least a 7% weight loss and at least 150 min of physical activity/week. The mean age of the participants was 51 years, and the mean BMI was 34 kg/m[2]; 68% were women, and 45% were members of minority groups. The average weight loss was 0.1, 2.1, and 5.6 kg in the placebo, metformin, and lifestyle-intervention groups, respectively. Thus, lifestyle modification was twice as effective as the drug in preventing type 2 diabetes in patients with abnormal glucose tolerance.

In another study[6] of 522 overweight Finnish men and women aged 55 years with average BMIs of 31 kg/m[2] and impaired glucose tolerance, *twice as many cases* of clinical type 2 diabetes were found in the control group (who did not receive any lifestyle counseling) compared to the lifestyle intervention group (who received individualized counseling aimed at reducing body weight and total intake of fat, especially saturated fat, and increasing intake of fiber and physical activity) (Fig. 14–5).

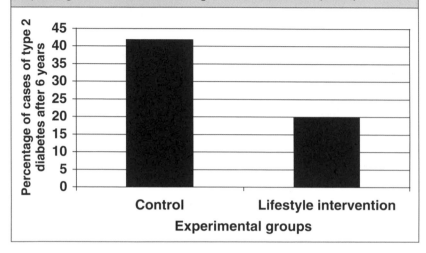

Figure 14–5. Lifestyle intervention in the form of physical activity and diet counseling reduced incidence of type 2 diabetes. (Adapted from Tuomilehto J, Lindstrom J, Eriksson JG, et al, Finnish Diabetes Prevention Study Group. Prevention of type 2 diabetes mellitus by changes in lifestyle among subjects with impaired glucose tolerance. New Engl J Med 344:1343–1350, 2001.)

Overweight/obese women who are in the lowest quartile of physical activity have a 40% higher risk of type 2 diabetes than overweight/obese women who are in the top two quartiles of physical activity (Fig. 14–6).[7] Note that overweight/obese women in the second lowest quartile of physical activity have a 20% reduction in the risk of having type 2 diabetes; these differences are clinically significant. Overweight patients have a much higher prevalence of type 2 diabetes than individuals with BMI < 25 kg/m². However, the decrease of type 2 diabetes in normal-weight *and* overweight individuals as physical activity increases demonstrates a dose-response effect of physical activity on type 2 diabetes that is *independent of body weight.*

Only moderate amounts of physical activity are necessary to produce health benefits. Physical activity is a valuable health measure for overweight patients. Obviously, the ideal is to prevent BMI > 25 kg/m² from ever occurring, but increasing physical activity levels regardless of body weight has tremendous health implications by significantly reducing the relative risk of type 2 diabetes.

Tertiary Prevention of Type 2 Diabetes Mellitus

A recent review from the Joslin Diabetes Center at Harvard University[8] concluded that the individual with type 2 diabetes can benefit from appropriate levels of physical activity and dietary intervention, and that the positive effects of physical activity include:

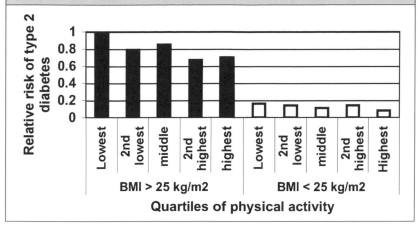

Figure 14–6. Physically active overweight patients have a lower risk of type 2 diabetes when compared to sedentary overweight individuals. (Data from Hu FB, Sigal RJ, Rich-Edwards JW, et al. Walking compared with vigorous physical activity and risk of type 2 diabetes in women: A prospective study. JAMA 282:1433–1439, 1999.)

- Increased energy expenditure
- Decreased body fat (particularly if combined with dietary restriction)
- Increased insulin sensitivity
- Improved long-term glycemic control
- Improved lipid profiles
- Lower blood pressure
- Increased cardiovascular fitness.

Another recent review[9] concluded that since most patients with diabetes die from complications of atherosclerosis, they should receive intensive preventive interventions proven to reduce their cardiovascular risk. Note that physicians should be careful in prescribing physical activity for patients with clinical type 2 diabetes. Patients may find it difficult to exercise and they are at increased risk for injury, exacerbation of underlying diseases, or metabolic complications. (See Chapter 8, "Physical Activity Prescription.")

Biochemical/Cellular Mechanisms

Glucose Uptake Pathways

How does physical activity signal skeletal muscle to take glucose from blood by a mechanism that does not use insulin? The insulin signaling pathway for glucose uptake by skeletal muscles in type 2 diabetes remains essentially dysfunctional both at rest and during physical activity.

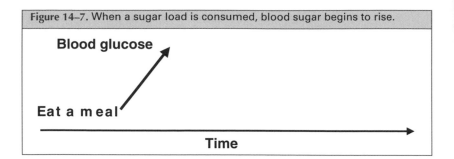

Figure 14–7. When a sugar load is consumed, blood sugar begins to rise.

Therefore, the contracting muscle takes up blood glucose by a pathway that is independent of insulin signaling. At least one other pathway signals skeletal muscle to take up glucose, independent of insulin signaling, and this explains the clinical observation made 50 years earlier that the dose of insulin has to be reduced when the diabetic patient exercises. The following figures (14–7 through 14–11) illustrate the pathway by which exercise stimulates glucose uptake independent of insulin.

Clearance of glucose from the blood to skeletal muscle in healthy individuals (Fig. 14–9):

- An individual without type 2 diabetes can use two signaling pathways to remove glucose from the blood into the muscle—via insulin receptor-mediated and physical activity–mediated translocation of the glucose carrier (GLUT4) to the muscle membrane.
- The importance of dual signaling is that blood insulin levels de-

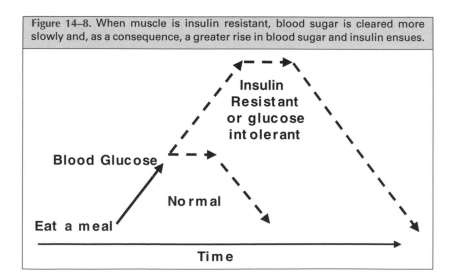

Figure 14–8. When muscle is insulin resistant, blood sugar is cleared more slowly and, as a consequence, a greater rise in blood sugar and insulin ensues.

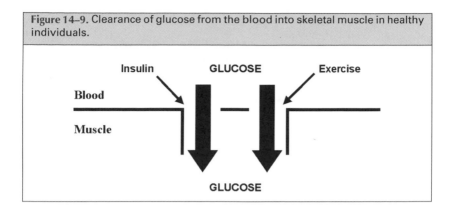

Figure 14–9. Clearance of glucose from the blood into skeletal muscle in healthy individuals.

cline with physical activity. Thus, insulin will not signal noncontracting skeletal muscles to take up blood glucose, hence conserving the blood glucose for those muscles that are contracting.
- A *localized* exercise signal in the contracting skeletal muscles selectively signals GLUT4 to the contracting muscle's plasma membrane so that blood glucose is only taken up by contracting muscles.

Clearance of glucose from the blood to skeletal muscle in patients with type 2 diabetes:
- Sedentary diabetic (Fig. 14–10)—The insulin signaling pathway is essentially inoperative in the diabetic skeletal muscle, and an inactive skeletal muscle has no exercise signal to stimulate the uptake of glucose from the blood.
- Physically active diabetic (Fig. 14–11)—Contracting skeletal muscles of the physically active individual with type 2 diabetes send a localized signal to move GLUT4 specifically to the contracting muscle membrane, thereby allowing the transport of glucose into the muscle cell even though the insulin signaling pathway is

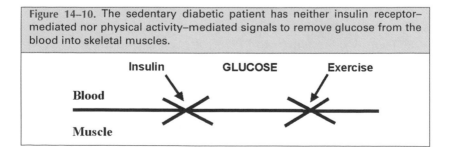

Figure 14–10. The sedentary diabetic patient has neither insulin receptor–mediated nor physical activity–mediated signals to remove glucose from the blood into skeletal muscles.

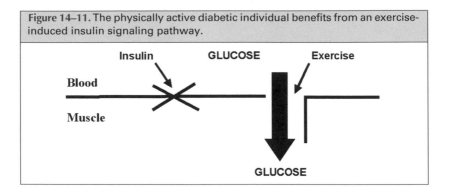

Figure 14–11. The physically active diabetic individual benefits from an exercise-induced insulin signaling pathway.

defective. The ability of localized muscle contraction to use a second signaling pathway to remove blood sugar explains why clinicians advise lowering the insulin dosage on days when patients with diabetes exercise.

Significance of Exercise-Induced Glucose Pathway

What is so important about exercise having its own signaling pathway to remove blood glucose? The insulin mechanism guides glucose from ingested food to tissues for storage. We described earlier (Chapters 1, 3, and 4) how evolution selected those functions that provided a survival advantage. During periods of feasting, insulin repletes glycogen stores (complexed glucose) in skeletal muscle and then in the liver. Once these glycogen stores are filled, insulin directs blood glucose into adipose tissue to be stored as fat. The "thrifty gene" hypothesis states that individuals with more efficient genes are able to store more of a given glucose meal as fat and are thus more likely to survive during famine.

The physical activity mechanism has two parts that likely evolved over 10,000 years ago as a survival advantage during the feast and famine cycles:

1. Physical activity signals the pancreas to markedly lower its release of insulin into the blood, thereby causing blood insulin concentration to fall. In famine, blood insulin concentrations are already low, so if our ancestors undertook physical activity in a hunt, they would not want their blood insulin to go to non-exercising tissues. Exercise (pursuit of food) would then have to stop due to the lack of glucose supply to the muscle. We speculate that alternative mechanisms were selected that allowed the exercising muscle to signal it to take up blood glucose when blood insulin was insufficient, i.e., independent of insulin. These ancient survival mechanisms are still present today, allowing the exercising diabetic muscle to efficiently take up and clear blood glucose.

2. The physical activity mechanism allows only contracting skeletal muscles to remove blood sugar by a localized process, thereby conserving limited blood glucose from non-contracting muscles. It was established in the 1930s that the running distance to exhaustion could be extended if blood glucose were not permitted to fall too low.[22]

The physical activity mechanism in the 21st century does not serve a famine purpose in societies where sedentary individuals have a continuous supply of food. Since our ancient genes require a certain threshold of physical activity for their physiological function, without this stimulus a sort of metabolic chaos results, described as dysfunction or pathophysiology. If all skeletal muscles are inactive, the whole body becomes insulin resistant in a few days, as skeletal muscle is responsible for 75–95% of the body's glucose clearance. As mentioned above, skeletal muscle is still genetically programmed to conserve blood glucose for a famine by shutting down its ability to take up blood glucose when inactive. Compounding the problem, blood glucose is not as low as during the feast and famine times of our ancestors, and is especially high due to reduced physical activity.

High blood levels of insulin in our ancestors helped store food as fat for the next famine by:

- Increasing the rate of VLDL formation in the liver
- Increasing the rate of cholesterol synthesis in liver
- Enhancing the uptake of triglyceride from the blood into adipose tissue and muscle
- Decreasing the rate of fatty acid oxidation in muscle and liver.

The same thrifty genes in our ancestors that efficiently stored food as fat now work continuously to accentuate the above metabolic changes in sedentary individuals predisposed to type 2 diabetes. Thus, physical activity is an absolute necessity to escape whole-body insulin resistance produced by inactive skeletal muscles.

Effects of a single bout of physical activity: The blood glucose and insulin are lowered after an oral glucose tolerance test (which is a surrogate for what happens after eating a meal) (Fig. 14–12). The clinical benefit is that post-meal hyperglycemia is less severe, and the magnitude of hyperinsulinemia is reduced. When blood glucose levels are lower, less insulin is signaled to be released from the pancreas.

Effects of repeated bouts of daily physical activity: The post-meal rise in blood glucose and insulin is lowered by slightly more than that seen after a single bout of physical activity of equal work intensity. The clinical significance of a physical activity-induced lowering of post-meal blood glucose and insulin is that they do not reach the post-meal levels seen in pre-diabetic and diabetic patients.

Effects of forced sedentariness: Enforced physical inactivity for 10

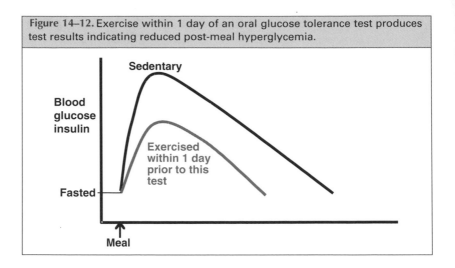

Figure 14–12. Exercise within 1 day of an oral glucose tolerance test produces test results indicating reduced post-meal hyperglycemia.

days in individuals previously exercising every day reverses the beneficial lowering of the post-meal rises in blood glucose and insulin (Fig. 14–13). Other studies have shown that this effect can occur in only 3 days of physical inactivity!

Restorative effects of even a single bout of physical activity: If physical activity is performed within 24 hours of ending 10 days of being sedentary, the beneficial effect of exercise training is regained (Fig. 14–14).[23] Thus, changes in insulin sensitivity in response to physical ac-

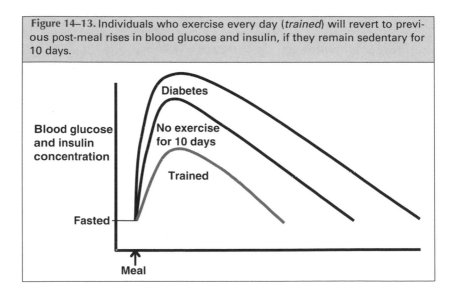

Figure 14–13. Individuals who exercise every day (*trained*) will revert to previous post-meal rises in blood glucose and insulin, if they remain sedentary for 10 days.

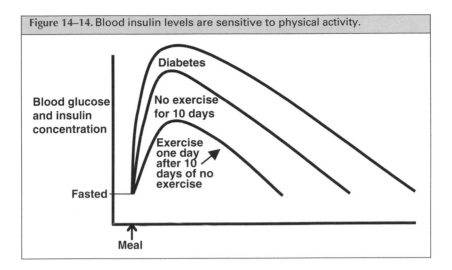

Figure 14–14. Blood insulin levels are sensitive to physical activity.

tivity occur rapidly, i.e., insulin sensitivity increases within 24 hours of an exercise bout and decreases within 2 days of the last exercise bout. The rapidity of this change probably offered survival to our hunter-gatherer ancestors by directing glucose just to the exercised muscles and lasting only long enough to replenish the muscle's depleted glycogen store, thereby ensuring a glucose supply to allow the next hunt for food.

Many potential mechanisms exist by which physical inactivity initiates skeletal muscle and, subsequently, whole body insulin resistance. Two of these are:

1. Elevation of plasma free fatty acid (FFA) levels, likely from abdominal adipose tissue, which in turn may inhibit insulin action at the peripheral target tissues such as skeletal muscle. This is supported by the fact that thiazolidinedione-mediated improvement in insulin sensitivity is triggered indirectly via a reduction in FFAs levels.

2. TNF-α and leptin may also cause insulin resistance.

Sensitivity of Blood Glucose Levels To Physical Activity

Skeletal muscle is the predominant site of insulin-dependent and non-insulin-dependent glucose disposal in humans. During hyperinsulinemia, insulin-mediated glucose uptake in skeletal muscle represents 75% and 95% of the body's rate of glucose clearance at euglycemia and hyperglycemia, respectively. The first detectable cellular defect in patients with type 2 diabetes is frequently the inability of skeletal muscle to respond to normal levels of circulating insulin. Insulin resistance is rapidly increased after a few days of physical inactivity.[24] Physical inactivity leads to prolonged periods of postprandial hyperglycemia and hyperinsulinemia.

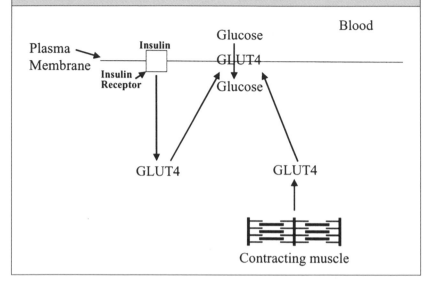

Figure 14–15. Insulin and muscle contraction can separately signal GLUT4 protein to move to the muscle cell membrane from separate storage sites within the muscle cell. At the muscle cell membrane, GLUT4 transfers blood glucose into the muscle cell.

These events are then analogous to the sequence of events leading to overt clinical type 2 diabetes.

Reduction in insulin action following short-term inactivity is the result of a decrease in insulin *sensitivity* (defined as a decrease in the concentration of insulin required to achieve a submaximal rate of glucose transport) and not a decrease in insulin *responsiveness*. Exercise increases insulin sensitivity because of increased number and activity of glucose transporters, both in muscle and adipose tissue. Long periods of inactivity are associated with a decreased insulin responsiveness, but not insulin sensitivity. The rate-limiting step in insulin- and exercise-induced glucose uptake is GLUT4 translocation to the cell membrane, where GLUT4 acts as a facilitated carrier of glucose into the cytoplasm from the extracellular space (Fig. 14–15).

Molecular Mechanisms

Signaling studies demonstrate that the underlying molecular mechanisms leading to the insulin- and physical activity–induced stimulation of glucose uptake in skeletal muscle are distinct. Winder and Hardie[10] first published that adenosine monophosphate kinase (AMPK) was activated in type IIa muscle fibers during treadmill running. Since then AMPK's role has been further delineated: it is a key energy-sensing/signaling protein of the skeletal muscle and has pleotropic effects. It is involved in:

Fatty acid oxidation
- AMPK phosphorylates and inactivates acetyl-CoA carboxylase, principally through the phosphorylation of serine 79.
- This phosphorylation event is a molecular switch to increase fatty acid oxidation during muscular contraction. It also limits fatty acid biosynthesis during times of ATP and glucose depletion.

GLUT4 (glucose carrier) translocation
- Contraction of skeletal muscle enhances membrane glucose transport capacity by recruiting GLUT4 to the sarcolemma and T-tubules. Exercise training increases the expression of GLUT4 in skeletal muscle.
- The activation of AMPK by adenosine analog 5-aminoimidazole-4-carboxamide-1-beta-D-ribofuranoside (AICAR) increases GLUT4 mRNA and protein expression in fast, but not slow, skeletal muscle.
- AICAR increases GLUT-4 mRNA through a transcriptional mechanism involving the interaction of myocyte enhancer factor-2 with 895 bp of the human GLUT-4 proximal promoter.

There are other mechanisms independent of either AMPK or insulin activation that enhance intracellular glucose uptake.[11] Moreover, there is also likely to be more than a single exercise-signaling pathway (Fig. 14–16). Physical activity increases the capacity of skeletal muscle to ox-

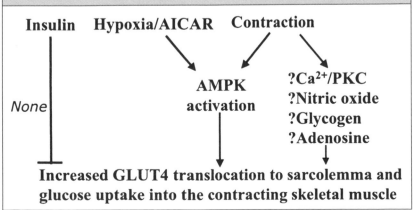

Figure 14–16. Other candidate signaling pathways by which localized muscle contraction could signal for GLUT4 to transport blood glucose into skeletal muscle. PKC = protein kinase C. (Adapted from Mu J, Brozinick JT Jr, Valladares O, et al: A role for AMP-activated protein kinase in contraction- and hypoxia-regulated glucose transport in skeletal muscle. Mol Cell 7:1085–1094, 2001.)

Insulin   Hypoxia/AICAR   Contraction

None

AMPK activation

?Ca²⁺/PKC
?Nitric oxide
?Glycogen
?Adenosine

Increased GLUT4 translocation to sarcolemma and glucose uptake into the contracting skeletal muscle

Figure 14–17. Daily physical activity maintains high levels of proteins involved with converting blood glucose and fatty acids to ATP. "Exercise" is a single bout of physical activity. "Training" is repeated bouts of exercise most days of the week leading to phenotypic changes. FFA = free fatty acids, LPL = lipoprotein lipase, IR = insulin receptor.

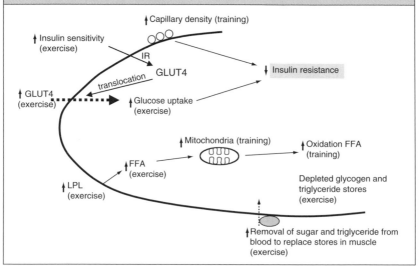

idize glucose and fatty acids (analogous to upsizing from a 4- to an 8-cylinder automobile; Fig. 14–17).

Obesity

Epidemiology

The CDC calls obesity an epidemic.[1] Each year, an estimated 300,000 adults die of causes related to obesity, making it the second greatest environmental cause of death after tobacco. Data for adults suggest that the overweight prevalence has increased by more than 50% in the last 10 years. An overweight condition is the most common health problem facing U.S. children, particularly among African Americans and Hispanics. The direct costs of obesity and physical inactivity accounted for 9.4% of U.S. healthcare expenditures more than 10 years ago, and must be greater now due to the doubling of obesity in this decade.

Effects of Physical Activity in the Obese

Beneficial effects of physical activity can occur independent of obesity. A review of the literature by Blair and Brodney[12] found that:
- Regular physical activity appeared to provide substantial protec-

tion against coronary heart disease (CHD), especially in over-weight men.

- Regular physical activity appears to reduce the risk of developing hypertension in men with elevated BMI, and this reduction was greatest in men in the high BMI categories.
- Physical fitness had the same protective effect in normal-weight diabetic men as overweight diabetic men.

Studies have demonstrated that weight loss is not necessary to benefit from the effects of physical activity on glucose tolerance and insulin sensitivity. *Inactive* women with BMIs < 29 kg/m^2 have a higher relative risk for CHD than *active* women with BMIs > 29 kg/m^2 (0.79 vs. 0.69).[25] Moderate-intensity aerobic training has a favorable effect on glucose tolerance in older people, independent of changes in abdominal adiposity.[26] These data suggest that the present emphasis on loss of body weight in overweight individuals, while appropriate, usually overlooks, in our opinion, the fact that inactivity—all by itself—worsens the prevalence of most chronic health conditions without a change in BMI. We further suggest that the health outcomes from campaigns to lower the number of calories consumed each day would be improved if a greater emphasis on moderate physical activity were included.

Primary Prevention of Obesity

The CDC had noted that the 300,000 deaths each year from obesity are largely preventable.[1] As a conservative approximation, we estimate that physical inactivity contributes to a minimum of 150,000 deaths (50%) from obesity each year in the U.S. Such an estimate is reasonable since some of the reports[13] imply, albeit wrongly in our opinion, that obesity is solely a "nutritional" disorder. (Please refer to Chapter 7, Caloric Balance and Expenditure).

In the UK, the rise in obesity from 1950 to 1990 was *not* associated with a change in caloric intake (Fig. 14–18).[14] This data strongly suggests that an increasingly sedentary lifestyle is linked to the increase in obesity.

Secondary Prevention

Secondary prevention focuses on avoiding additional gain in body weight. Check the chart records of patients approaching overweight (BMI in 75th–85th percentile for gender in children/adolescents and BMI 24–25 kg/m^2 in adults) to determine if their percentile rank or BMI has been holding steady or even decreasing over the past few years. If BMI or rank has held steady or decreased, then the parent/child and the adult should be congratulated, and maintenance counseling can be initiated. However, if the charts indicate a rise, then secondary prevention must be initiated (see Chapters 9 and 10 for details).

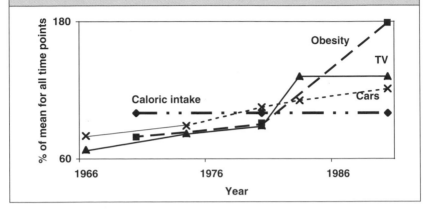

Figure 14–18. An increased rate of obesity (*squares*) was associated with an increase in both the number of hours of TV viewing (*triangles*) and the number of cars per household (*X*). It was not associated with a change in caloric intake (*diamonds*). (Data from Prentice AM, Jebb SA: Obesity in Britain: Gluttony or sloth? BMJ 311:437–439, 1995.)

Tertiary Prevention

Tertiary prevention centers on permanent loss of body fat. Individuals who combine caloric restriction and exercise with behavioral treatment may expect to lose about 5–10% of pre-intervention body weight over a period of 4–6 months.[13] Such decreases are clinically significant. Small decreases in BMI in patients with BMIs > 25 kg/m^2 can reduce death rates from numerous comorbidities.

Biochemical/Cellular Mechanisms

Physically active subjects have smaller adipose tissue stores. Biochemical changes favoring a smaller steady-state size of adipose tissue during physical activity are increased fat oxidation and adrenergic stimulation of lipolysis (Fig. 14–19). Additional factors, such as increased TNF-α and decreased leptin, may play roles.

Blood catecholamine levels increase less in the trained state than in the sedentary state at the same absolute workload. Fat cells appear to become more sensitive to catecholamines, resulting in the activation of the lipolytic β-adrenergic pathway in subcutaneous abdominal adipose tissues. Since one of the consequences of exercise training is decreased adipose tissue mass, one might expect leptin concentrations would be decreased, which was indeed the case in insulin-resistant rats that voluntarily ran on exercise wheels, compared to sedentary rats.[27] Such decreases in leptin concentrations could negatively feedback to oppose the training-associated decrease. For example, acute adiposity-independent

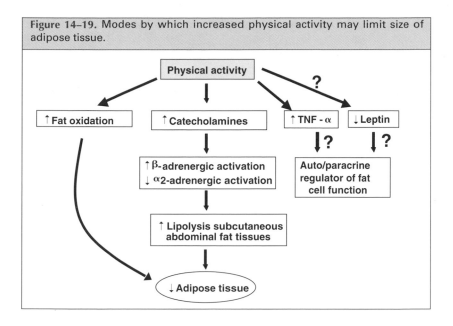

Figure 14–19. Modes by which increased physical activity may limit size of adipose tissue.

decreases of leptin production in response to an energy deficit in non-exercise situations have been shown to promote increased energy intake and energy conservation before body fat stores become significantly depleted.[28] However, human studies report mixed changes in blood leptin levels with exercise training, and it is presently unclear if leptin regulates fat cells to ultimately decrease fat mass.

Cytokines such as TNF-α were also shown to be elevated in adipose tissues of rats that voluntarily exercised, and are hypothesized to function as autocrine/paracrine regulators in fat cells, limiting adipose tissue expansion by as yet unknown mechanisms. Increases in serum TNF-α have also been noted after physical exertion in humans.

While exercise training increases fat oxidation in lean individuals, the capacity to mobilize and oxidize fat may be impaired in obese individuals.[15] This could be one of the reasons it is so difficult for most obese individuals to attain a BMI ≤ 25 kg/m².

Dyslipidemia

Epidemiology

Physical inactivity in 51 studies involving 4700 subjects[29] showed the following patterns:

- Decreased plasma HDL-C by 4.4%, which represents an

approximate increase in coronary heart disease risk of 4% in men and 6% in women.

- Increased plasma triglycerides, LDL-C, and total cholesterol by 3.8%, 5.3%, and 1.0%, respectively.

The effect of physical activity is most pronounced postprandially, but the effect is missed clinically.[16] Blood lipids must be measured in the fasting state so that the results can be compared to population norms. Otherwise, patients would present with huge postprandial variations in lipid levels related to the timing and content of their last meal, and meaningful diagnosis would be impossible. Note, however, that fasting is not a natural condition for most individuals in the U.S. On a population basis, repeated elevations of postprandial triglyceride-rich lipoproteins do contribute to the development of atherosclerosis/CHD. Unfortunately, the role of physical activity on blood lipids is underestimated due to the testing procedures.

Biochemical and Cellular Mechanisms

A single preceding bout of exercise decreases the rise in post-meal blood lipids (i.e., diminishes postprandial hyperlipidemia). The rise in blood triglycerides is attenuated after a high-fat, high-carbohydrate meal if an aerobic (treadmill run or walk) bout of exercise preceded the meal by 16–18 hours in untrained women (Fig. 14–20).[16]

In another report,[17] reductions of 28%, 42%, and 45% in the post-meal rise in blood total triglycerides, VLDL-triglycerides, and chylomicron-triglycrides, respectively, were produced by physical activity (2 hrs at 60% of maximal effort running on a motor-driven treadmill) that had been performed 16 hours prior to eating a fatty meal at time zero in men. The clinical significance of post-exercise–induced reductions in plasma triglycerides is that most sedentary individuals in the U.S. are likely "persistently" hyperlipidemic, considering the relatively brief, perhaps even nonexistent periods of true fasting during a 24-hour period. As the exercise-induced reduction in plasma triglycerides is greater after a meal than in a fast, the true significance of the exercise-induced reduction of plasma lipids is likely underestimated. There are two mechanisms by which physical activity attenuates the rise in blood triglycerides after a fatty meal:

1. Increased clearance of triglycerides from the blood by the previously exercised skeletal muscle (Fig. 14–21)

2. Increased lipoprotein lipase (LPL) activity in exercising skeletal muscles

- LPL activity in the blood and skeletal muscle peaks about 4 to 18 hours post-exercise as it takes this long for LPL to increase in the

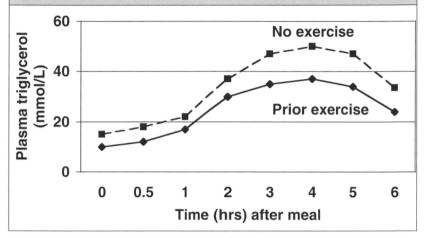

Figure 14–20. Untrained women engaged in aerobic exercise 16 hours before consuming 1.7 g fat, 1.65 g carbohydrate, and 0.25 g protein/kg of body mass (*point before time zero on x axis*). Note the significant attenuation in the post-meal rise in plasma triglycerides in the "prior exercise" group, compared to the "no exercise" group. (Adapted from Gill JM, Hardman AE. Postprandial lipemia: Effects of exercise and restriction of energy intake compared. Am J Clin Nutr 71:465–471, 2000.)

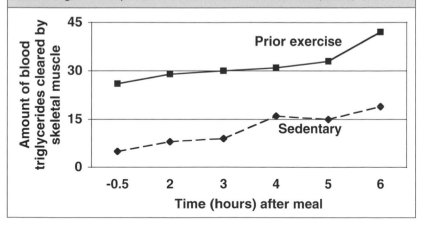

Figure 14–21. Skeletal muscles of individuals who exercised 16 hours prior to the ingestion of a high-fat meal removed (cleared) 3.5 times more of the blood triglycerides than of sedentary subjects. (Adapted from Malkova D, Evans RD, Frayn KN, et al: Prior exercise and postprandial substrate extraction across the human leg. Am J Physiol Endocrinol Metab 279:E1020–1028, 2000.)

capillaries of the exercised muscles. Postprandial plasma triglycerides peak about 4 hours after a meal.

- Individuals with the lowest LPL activity in skeletal muscles after exercise also had the highest increases in postprandial hyperlipidemia.

Blood HDL-C increased the most after exercise if the exercise bout had been performed 12 hours prior to the meal (Fig 14–22).[18] The increase in HDL-C was associated with an increase in LPL activity. Increased levels of HDL-C are seen in the venous blood from exercising skeletal muscles.

The effect of a single bout of physical activity in lowering the post-meal hyperlipidemia is short-lived, and thus is of clinical significance (Fig. 14–23). Persistent, routine physical activity is required to obtain and maintain the benefits of the lipid-lowering effects of physical activity.

Physical activity increases LPL activity in skeletal muscle, allowing the muscle to take up and replenish its stores of triglycerides (Fig. 14–24). Initial changes in LPL levels in fat and skeletal muscle are mediated via post-translational mechanisms. Concurrently, the transcription rate of the LPL gene has been reported to be lower in the non-exercising leg muscle as compared to muscle recovering from 60–90 minutes of exhaustive one-legged knee extensor exercises. The signaling mechanisms by which physical inactivity keeps skeletal muscle LPL low are unknown. However, it is known that physical activity increases skeletal muscle LPL pro-

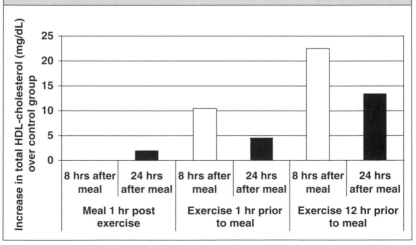

Figure 14–22. Optimal timing of meal to achieve increased HDL-C post-exercise. The exercise bout consisted of men running for 1 hour at 60% of maximal aerobic capacity. (Adapted from Zhang JQ, Thomas TR, Ball SD: Effect of exercise timing on postprandial lipidemia and HDL cholesterol subfractions. J Appl Physiol 85:1516–1522, 1998.)

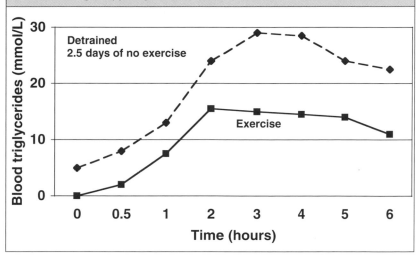

Figure 14–23. Improved fat tolerance was lost in previously trained subjects after only 2.5 days of no exercise. (Adapted from Hardman AE, Lawrence JE, Herd SL. Postprandial lipemia in endurance-trained people during a short interruption to training. J Appl Physiol 84:1895–1901, 1998.)

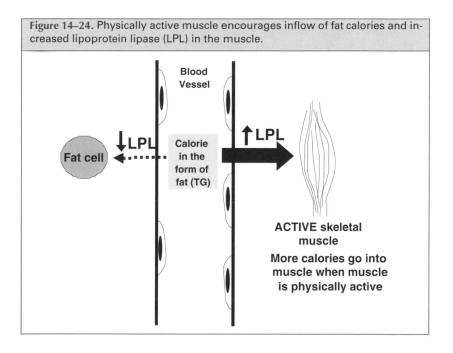

Figure 14–24. Physically active muscle encourages inflow of fat calories and increased lipoprotein lipase (LPL) in the muscle.

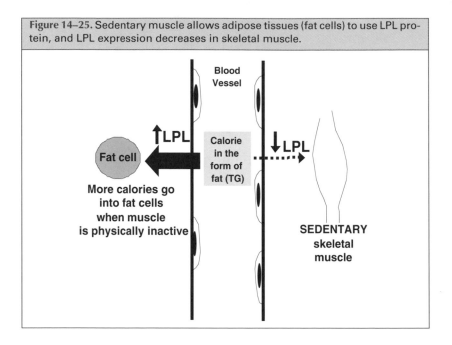

Figure 14–25. Sedentary muscle allows adipose tissues (fat cells) to use LPL protein, and LPL expression decreases in skeletal muscle.

tein content via alterations in local cellular homeostasis, rather than by adrenergic-receptor stimulation.

Physical inactivity (sedentary state) results in a preferential uptake of fat or sugar into adipose tissues, rather than skeletal muscle (Fig. 14–25). The preferential upregulation of LPL protein in fat cells by physical inactivity causes the breakdown of triglycerides in capillaries around fat cells, which directs blood fat into fat cells. Furthermore, physical inactivity decreases the expression of LPL protein in skeletal muscles. Consequently, triglyceride breakdown is minimized in capillaries supplying skeletal muscle.

Gallbladder Disease

Epidemiology

Chuang et al[20] demonstrated that low levels of physical activity are associated with gallstone formation. Sedentary behavior, as assessed by time spent sitting, was positively correlated with the risk of cholecystectomy in a prospective study of 60,290 women. In the same study, an average of 2 to 3 hours of recreational exercise per week appeared to reduce the risk of cholecystectomy by approximately 20%.

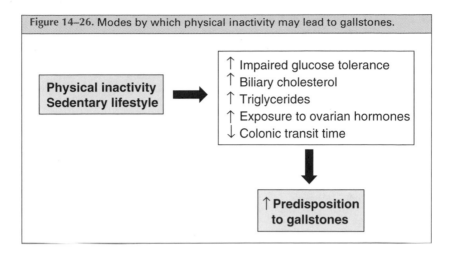

Figure 14–26. Modes by which physical inactivity may lead to gallstones.

Biochemical and Cellular Mechanisms

Leitzmann et al[21] speculated that there are probably several metabolic pathways by which physical inactivity may increase the risk of gallstone disease, *independent* of the effect of physical inactivity on body weight (Fig. 14–26). Furthermore, physical inactivity by itself is a plausible cause of gallstones because its metabolic consequences, including insulin resistance and hyperinsulinemia, are similar to those of obesity.

Suggested Reading

1. Mokdad AH, Bowman BA, Ford ES, et al. The continuing epidemics of obesity and diabetes in the United States. JAMA 286: 1195–1200, 2001.
2. Hu FB, Manson JE, Stampfer MJ, et al. Diet, lifestyle, and the risk of type 2 diabetes mellitus in women. New Engl J Med 345: 790–797, 2001.
3. Certain LK, Kahn RS. Prevalence, correlates, and trajectory of television viewing among infants and toddlers. Pediatrics 109(4):634–642, 2002.
4. Hu FB, Leitzmann MF, Stampfer MJ, et al. Physical activity and television watching in relation to risk for type 2 diabetes mellitus in men. Arch Intern Med 161:1542–1548, 2001.
5. Knowler WC, Barrett-Connor E, Fowler SE, et al; Diabetes Prevention Program Research Group. Reduction in the incidence of type 2 diabetes with lifestyle intervention or metformin. New Engl J Med 346:393–403, 2002.
6. Tuomilehto J, Lindstrom J, Eriksson JG, et al; Finnish Diabetes Prevention Study Group. Prevention of type 2 diabetes mellitus by changes in lifestyle among subjects with impaired glucose tolerance. New Engl J Med 344:1343–1350, 2001.
7. Hu FB, Sigal RJ, Rich-Edwards JW, et al. Walking compared with vigorous physical activity and risk of type 2 diabetes in women: A prospective study. JAMA 282:1433–1439, 1999.

8.   Hamdy O, Goodyear LJ, Horton ES. Diet and exercise in type 2 diabetes mellitus. Endocrinol Metab Clin North Am 30:883–907, 2001.
9.   Beckman JA, Creager MA, Libby P. Diabetes and atherosclerosis: Epidemiology, pathophysiology, and management. JAMA 287:2570–2581, 2002.
10. Winder WW, Hardie DG. Inactivation of acetyl-CoA carboxylase and activation of AMP-activated protein kinase in muscle during exercise. Am J Physiol Endocrinol Metab 270: E299–E304, 1996.
11. Mu J, Brozinick JT Jr, Valladares O, et al. A role for AMP-activated protein kinase in contraction- and hypoxia-regulated glucose transport in skeletal muscle. Mol Cell 7:1085–1094, 2001.
12. Blair SN, Brodney S. Effects of physical inactivity and obesity on morbidity and mortality: Current evidence and research issues. Med Sci Sports Exerc 31: S646–S662, 1999.
13. Yanovski SZ, Yanovski JA. Obesity. N Engl J Med 346:591–602, 2002.
14. Prentice AM, Jebb SA. Obesity in Britain: Gluttony or sloth? BMJ 311:437–439, 1995.
15. van Baak MA. Exercise training and substrate utilisation in obesity. Int J Obes Relat Metab Disord 23 Suppl 3:S11–S17, 1999.
16. Gill JM, Hardman AE. Postprandial lipemia: Effects of exercise and restriction of energy intake compared. Am J Clin Nutr 71:465–471, 2000.
17. Malkova D, Evans RD, Frayn KN, et al. Prior exercise and postprandial substrate extraction across the human leg. Am J Physiol Endocrinol Metab 279:E1020–1028, 2000.
18. Zhang JQ, Thomas TR, Ball SD. Effect of exercise timing on postprandial lipemia and HDL cholesterol subfractions. J Appl Physiol 85:1516–1522, 1998.
19. Hardman AE, Lawrence JE, Herd SL. Postprandial lipemia in endurance-trained people during a short interruption to training. J Appl Physiol 84:1895–1901, 1998.
20. Chuang CZ, Martin LF, LeGardeur BY, Lopez A. Physical activity, biliary lipids, and gallstones in obese subjects. Am J Gastroenterol 96: 1860–1865, 2001.
21. Leitzmann MF, Rimm EB, Willett WC, et al. Recreational physical activity and the risk of cholecystectomy in women. New Engl J Med 341: 777–784, 1999.
22. Christensen EH, Hansen O. Arbeits Fähigkeit und Ehrnährung. Skand Arch Physiol 81:160, 1939.
23. Heath GW, Gavin JR III, Hinderliter JM, et al. Effects of exercise and lack of exercise on glucose tolerance and insulin sensitivity. J Appl Physiol 55:512–517, 1983.
24. Smorawinski J, Kaciuba-Uscillo H, Nazar K, et al. Effects of three-day bed rest on metabolic, hormonal, and circulatory responses to an oral glucose load on endurance or strength trained athletes and untrained subjects. J Physiol Pharmacol 51: 279–289, 2000.
25. Manson JE, Hu F, Rich-Edwards JW, et al. A prospective study of walking as compared with vigorous exercise in the prevention of coronary heart disease in women. New Engl J Med 341:650–658, 1999.
26. DiPietro L, Seeman TE, Stachenfeld NS, et al. Moderate-intensity aerobic training improves glucose tolerance in aging independent of abdominal adiposity. J Am Geriatr Soc 46:875–879, 1998.
27. Nara M, Kanda T, Tsukui S, et al. Reduction of leptin precedes fat loss from running exercise in insulin-resistant rats. Exp Clin Endocrinol Diabetes 107:431–434, 1999.
28. Jequier E. Leptin signaling, adiposity, and energy balance. Ann NY Acad Sci 967: 379–388, 2002.
29. Leon AS, Sanchez OA. Response of blood lipids to exercise training alone or combined with dietary intervention. Med Sci Sports Exerc 33 Suppl 6:S502–S515, 2001.

Cancer

chapter
15

Overview

In a study examining cancer causation in twin cohorts from Sweden, Denmark, and Finland, Lichtenstein et al[1] concluded that the majority of sporadic cancers were indeed caused by environmental factors, including physical inactivity (Fig. 15–1). The genetic component contributed only to a minor degree. In all cases, the environmental factors predominated over the heritable factors in causing the many types of cancers.

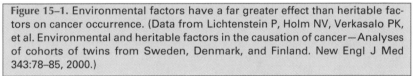

Figure 15–1. Environmental factors have a far greater effect than heritable factors on cancer occurrence. (Data from Lichtenstein P, Holm NV, Verkasalo PK, et al. Environmental and heritable factors in the causation of cancer—Analyses of cohorts of twins from Sweden, Denmark, and Finland. New Engl J Med 343:78–85, 2000.)

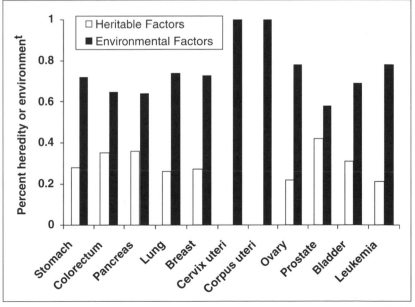

This chapter provides specific evidence for the role(s) of physical inactivity as an important environmental factor contributing to the causation of many, but not all, cancers. The American Cancer Society (ACS) states that one-third of the more than 500,000 cancer deaths that occur in the United States each year can be attributed to diet and physical activity habits, with another third due to cigarette smoking. Our conservative calculations (see following pages) indicate that at least 34,000 premature cancer deaths occur each year in the U.S. due to physical inactivity. The ACS has issued guidelines on nutrition and physical activity for cancer prevention (Table 1).

Colon Cancer

Epidemiology

The colon is the third most common site of cancer, after the lung and breast. The American Cancer Society estimates that there will be 107,300 new cases of colon cancer and 48,100 deaths from this disease in 2002. The Harvard Report on Cancer[2] concluded that physical inactivity was the environmental risk factor most consistently shown to be associated with an increased risk of colon cancer. Remarkably, observations across numerous studies have shown that individuals at the highest level of physical activity have a 50% reduction in the incidence of colon cancer, and those who are sedentary have twice the incidence of colon cancer as compared to these individuals.[6]

Physical activity is more powerful than any drug (there being none) to *primarily prevent* the third most prevalent cancer. We estimate that 18,935 premature colon cancer cases and 8488 deaths are *already prevented* in those 30% of individuals who are more physically active than the U.S. Surgeon General's recommended 30 minutes of moderate activity each day. An additional 44,182 premature cases and 19,806 premature deaths from colon cancer could be prevented each year if the remaining 70% of sedentary individuals undertook high levels of physical activity each day.

TABLE 1. American Cancer Society Guideline on Physical Activity for Cancer Prevention, 2002

Adults:
- Engage in at least 30 min or more of moderate activity on 5 or more days/wk.
- Moderate-to-vigorous activity for 45 min or more on 5 or more days/wk may further enhance reductions in the risk of breast and colon cancer.

Children and adolescents:
- Engage in at least 60 min/day of moderate-to-vigorous physical activity for at least 5 days/wk.

Biochemical/Cellular Mechanisms

Men at low levels of physical activity were more likely than women at the same low levels to have a tumor with a Kirsten-ras (K-*ras*) mutation.[7] On the other hand, women with a higher BMI were more likely to have a K-ras mutation in their tumor. Mutations in the K-ras gene are associated with 30–50% of colon tumors and are thought to follow the initiation of the neoplastic process by an earlier mutation in the adenomatous polyposis coli (APC) gene (Fig. 15–2).

Pancreatic Cancer

Epidemiology

Walking or hiking < 20 min/wk was associated with twice the risk of pancreatic cancer when compared with ≥ 4 hrs/wk in 164,000 men and women.[3] Among non-overweight participants (BMI < 25 kg/m²) in this study, total physical activity was not related to the risk of pancreatic cancer. However, total physical activity was inversely associated with risk among overweight individuals.

The American Cancer Society estimates total pancreatic cancer cases

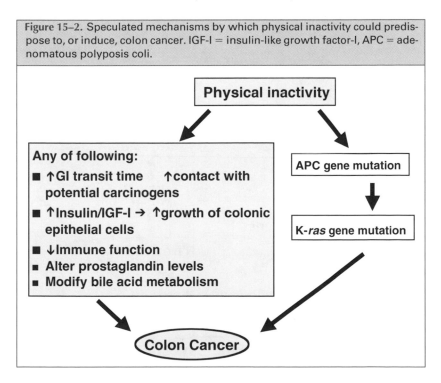

Figure 15–2. Speculated mechanisms by which physical inactivity could predispose to, or induce, colon cancer. IGF-I = insulin-like growth factor-I, APC = adenomatous polyposis coli.

and deaths in 2002 to be 30,300 and 29,700, respectively. Based on the information above, we estimate that the 30% of the U.S. population that undertakes 30 minutes of moderate physical activity each day is already preventing 2937 premature deaths and 2997 cases of pancreatic cancer each year. If the 70% of the sedentary population undertook walking 30 minutes or more each day for 5 or more days per week, then up to 6992 additional premature cases and 6854 premature deaths would be prevented. No known pharmaceutical approach achieves such potent prevention!

Biochemical/Cellular Mechanisms

Michaud et al[3] speculated that their findings of physical inactivity's contribution to increased pancreatic cancer in subjects with BMI > 25 kg/m^2 could be explained by high postprandial plasma glucose levels and hyperinsulinemia, ultimately resulting in increased free insulin-like growth factor-I (IGF-I). IGF-I has been shown to promote growth in human pancreatic cell lines (Fig. 15–3). Currently, little information is available describing cellular mechanisms.

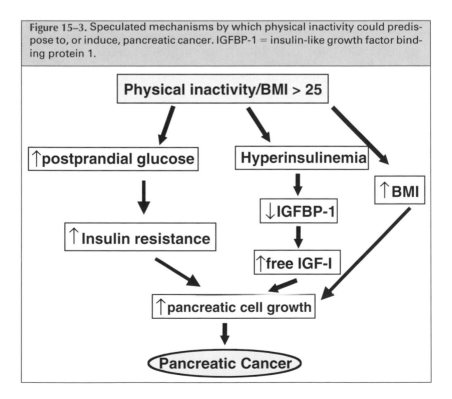

Figure 15–3. Speculated mechanisms by which physical inactivity could predispose to, or induce, pancreatic cancer. IGFBP-1 = insulin-like growth factor binding protein 1.

Melanoma

Epidemiology

Sedentary men and women had a 56% and 72%, respectively, higher incidence of melanomas than those exercising 5–7 days/wk.[4] Exercising ≤ 4 days/wk provided no protection from melanomas. For 2002, the American Cancer Society estimates total melanoma cases to be 58,300 and deaths to be 9600. Based on this information, we estimate that if the 70% of the sedentary population were to undertake moderate-intensity physical activity 5 or more days per week, then up to 13,454 premature cases and 2215 premature deaths could be additionally prevented.

Biochemical/Cellular Mechanisms

Shors et al[4] state that the mechanisms for the effect of exercise are unknown, but they suggest several avenues for additional research of the physical inactivity–melanoma association (Fig. 15–4), including:

- Various metabolic effects which may arise from inactivity, such as hormonal effects and depressed immune function
- Inactivity-induced increases in BMI, as an increased body weight has been shown to explain some, but not all, of the exercise effect on melanoma risk.

Currently, little information is available describing cellular mechanisms.

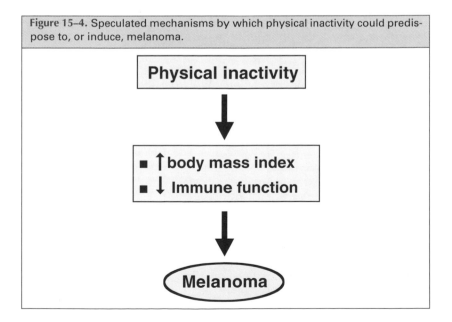

Figure 15–4. Speculated mechanisms by which physical inactivity could predispose to, or induce, melanoma.

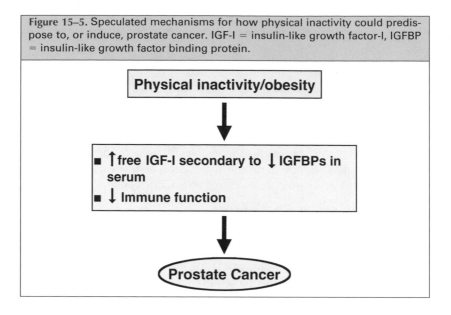

Figure 15–5. Speculated mechanisms for how physical inactivity could predispose to, or induce, prostate cancer. IGF-I = insulin-like growth factor-I, IGFBP = insulin-like growth factor binding protein.

Prostate Cancer

Epidemiology

Epidemiological data supporting the hypothesis that physical inactivity increases the incidence of prostrate cancer is weak and inconsistent. Therefore, additional studies are needed to clarify whether physical activity plays a role in the prevention of prostrate cancer.

Biochemical/Cellular Mechanisms

However, there is evidence at the cellular level (Fig. 15–5) that physical inactivity does increase the growth of prostate cells, in cell culture models. Tymchuk et al[5] found that the application of serum from men who had been on a low-fat, high-fiber diet and exercising for 11 days reduced the growth of androgen dependent LNCaP prostate cells in culture by 30%, compared to the serum applied from pre-lifestyle modifications. The factor in the serum remains to be identified.

Key Points

⇨ The American Cancer Society estimates that there are currently a total of 1,284,900 cancer cases and 555,000 cancer deaths annually in the U.S.

Key Points (*Continued*)

☞ Moderate-to-vigorous levels of physical activity ≥ 30 min/day on 5 or more days/wk can prevent up to 86,500 of these cases (~7%) and 34,000 of these deaths from cancer (~6%).

☞ Currently, there is no drug for primary prevention that can make this claim.

Suggested Reading

1. Lichtenstein P, Holm NV, Verkasalo PK, et al. Environmental and heritable factors in the causation of cancer—Analyses of cohorts of twins from Sweden, Denmark, and Finland. New Engl J Med 343:78–85, 2000.

2. Tomeo CA, Colditz GA, Willett WC, et al. Harvard Report on Cancer Prevention. Volume 3: Prevention of colon cancer in the United States. Cancer Causes Control 10: 167–180, 1999.

3. Michaud DS, Giovannucci E, Willett WC, et al. Physical activity, obesity, height, and the risk of pancreatic cancer. JAMA 286: 921–929, 2001.

4. Shors AR, Solomon C, McTiernan A, White E. Melanoma risk in relation to height, weight, and exercise (United States). Cancer Causes Control 12: 599–606, 2001.

5. Tymchuk CN, Barnard RJ, Heber D, Aronson WJ. Evidence of an inhibitory effect of diet and exercise on prostate cancer cell growth. J Urol 166: 1185–1189, 2001.

6. Thune I, Furberg AS. Physical activity and cancer risk: Dose-response and cancer, all sites and site-specific. Med Sci Sports Exerc 33(6 Suppl) S530–S550, 2001.

7. Slattery ML, Anderson K, Curtin K, et al. Lifestyle factors and K-*ras* mutations in colon cancer tumors. Mutat Res 483:73–81, 2001.

Aging

chapter

16

Epidemiology of Aging

Both the proportion of the U.S. population and the absolute number of individuals who are older than 65 years are increasing (Fig. 16–1). Thus, many of the aging-associated changes in multiple body functions (i.e., decline in **functional capacity**) will become more widespread in the U.S. population. Decline in functional capacity with aging often leads to **"physical frailty,"** a condition of failure to thrive or weakness. Increasingly, the term physical frailty is used to describe combinations of aging, disease, and other factors (e.g., fitness, nutritional status) that make some people more *susceptible to* decreased functional capacity.

Functional capacity relates to both skeletal muscle and aerobic capacity. Loss of the functional capacity of **skeletal muscle** with aging leads to physical frailty. The individual finds it difficult or impossible to perform

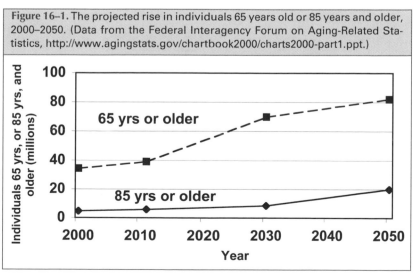

Figure 16–1. The projected rise in individuals 65 years old or 85 years and older, 2000–2050. (Data from the Federal Interagency Forum on Aging-Related Statistics, http://www.agingstats.gov/chartbook2000/charts2000-part1.ppt.)

225

activities of daily living, such as having enough leg strength to rise from a toilet. Muscle mass and strength have declined.

Loss of the functional capacity of **aerobic work** with aging means that an aerobic task that was non-fatiguing at the age of 20 years becomes tiring very quickly at the age of 70 years. For example, the same intensity of aerobic work requires the same number of calories at the ages of 20 and 70 years (assuming body mass is the same). However, due to the drop in the maximal number of calories that can be expended per minute in the 70-year-old, the older person may be working at 80% of his or her maximal aerobic capacity; the same work may have required only 40% maximal capacity at age 20. Since work time to fatigue decreases as the percentage of work done at maximal aerobic capacity increases, the 70-year-old can't work as long as he or she did at 50. As a consequence, the elderly tend to eliminate many physical activity tasks, which sets up a vicious negative cycle: the more tasks eliminated, the greater the sedentary lifestyle, and the faster the functional capacity declines (Fig. 16–2).

Remarkably, a physically active lifestyle delays this decline in the functional capacity of many organ systems with aging, as attested by the following statements:

"A review of biologic changes commonly attributed to the process of aging demonstrates the close similarity of most of these to changes subsequent to a period of enforced physical inactivity. The coincidence of these changes from subcellular to whole-body level of organization, and across a wide range of body systems, prompts the suggestion that at least a portion of the changes that

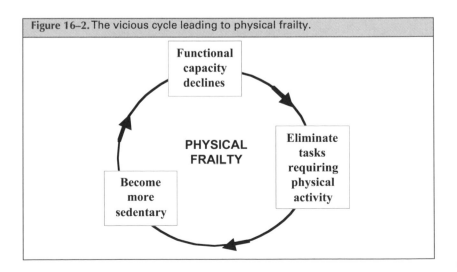

Figure 16–2. The vicious cycle leading to physical frailty.

are commonly attributed to aging is in reality caused by disuse, and as such, is subject to correction. There is no drug in current or prospective use that holds as much promise for sustained health as a lifetime of physical exercise."[1]

"While hunter-gatherers and other people who continue critical aspects of the Paleolithic life experience undergo age-related bodily deterioration as do Westerners—albeit, in some respects (vision, hearing) more slowly—their overall health pattern is quite different. With the exception of osteoporosis, they rarely develop 'chronic degenerative diseases.' Biomarkers of incipient illness such as rising blood pressure, increasing adiposity, deficient lean body mass, hypercholesterolemia, nonocclusive atheromata, and insulin resistance are quite infrequent among foragers and other similar traditional peoples compared with their prevalence in similar-aged Western populations. These observations suggest that many chronic degenerative disorders are not unavoidable concomitants of aging, but conditions that develop frequently when behavioral and environmental circumstances differ from those which our ancestors evolved."[2]

"Much can be done to prevent the progression and even the onset of disease in older people . . . Exercise should be encouraged not only because of its beneficial effects on blood pressure, cardiovascular conditioning, glucose homeostasis, bone density, and functional status, but also because it may improve mood and social interaction, reduce insomnia and constipation, and prevent falls."[3]

Thus, as a general rule, physical inactivity not only accelerates the process of aging-associated decline in the functional capacity of many organ systems, but it also mimics many of the changes associated with aging! In striking contrast, physical activity not only delays decline but maintains functional capacity at higher levels, thereby staving off many age-associated clinical disorders.

In a comprehensive review of the literature, Spirduso and Cronin[4] concluded that regular physical activity and physical disability are inversely related, i.e., physical inactivity predicts frailty and health-related disability. Older adults with chronic diseases experience a long-term beneficial mortality effect from participation in physical activity programs.[27] Another literature review of 31 studies[5] summarized that the most consistent positive effects of late-life exercise were improved strength, aerobic capacity, flexibility, walking, and standing balance.

Many scientists have overlooked the molecular processes and the biological significance of physical activity in delaying aging-associated decline in multiple body functions. In this chapter, we show how physical activity delays changes that are attributed to aging and delineate the currently known molecular mechanisms underlying some of these changes. We discuss the effects of physical inactivity/activity on several major systems (Table 16–1).

Skeletal Muscle Mass, Strength, and Balance

Physical activity delays the decline in skeletal muscle mass, strength, and balance with aging. Conversely, physical *inactivity* speeds the loss of skeletal muscle strength and thus the onset of physical frailty during aging (Fig. 16–3). Aging and physical inactivity *independently* cause a loss in muscle strength. Resistance training in the elderly, if performed regularly for the rest of their lives, can indeed slow the decline in muscle strength.

Increased mortality occurs when skeletal muscle mass falls below a threshold. For example, when body cell masses declined below 60% of normal levels for young adults, death was certain. This observation was first made by Krieger,[6] and later more comprehensively and tragically by the Warsaw Ghetto investigators.[7] It has been upheld in modern studies of patients with AIDS. Similarly, it was found in the Cardiovascular Health Study that individuals who had lost 10% or more of their body weight after age 50 had a relatively high death rate.[8] When that group was excluded, there was no remaining relationship between BMI and mortality.

Risk of mortality is statistically increased for both men and women who have lost 10% or more of their maximum lifetime weight within the last 10 years, even when controlling for current weight.[9] An inverse association of weight and mortality in old age appeared to reflect illness-

Organ System/Marker	Effects of Physical *Inactivity* On Symptoms of Aging	Effects of Physical Activity On Symptoms of Aging
TABLE 16–1.	**Effects of Physical Inactivity/Activity On Aging**	
Physical frailty	Onset accelerated	Onset delayed
Skeletal muscle strength	Decline accelerated	Decline slowed
Maximal aerobic capacity	Decline accelerated	Decline slowed
Insulin resistance	Increase accelerated	Almost completely prevented with sufficient activity
Cognitive impairment/ dysfunction	Accelerated in 2 of 4 studies	Impairment reduced in 2 of 4 studies
Bone mass	Reduction accelerated	Reduction prevented with sufficient activity

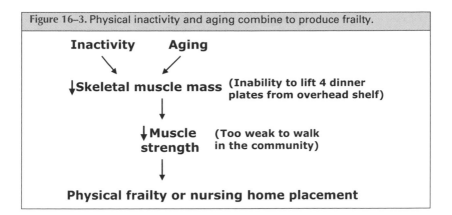

Figure 16–3. Physical inactivity and aging combine to produce frailty.

Inactivity   Aging

↓Skeletal muscle mass   (Inability to lift 4 dinner
                        plates from overhead shelf)

↓Muscle   (Too weak to walk
strength   in the community)

Physical frailty or nursing home placement

related weight loss from heavier weight in middle-age. Thus, either large amounts or increased rates in the decline of muscle mass are associated with increased mortality.

Decline in muscle mass and strength with aging can be counteracted by physical activity. Morganti et al found that 60-year-old women gained strength in three muscle groups after 12 months of resistance exercise training, thus slowing the rate of decline in muscle strength with aging (Fig. 16–4).[10] Moreover, strength gains occurred throughout the year of training (Fig. 16–5). As the load was continuously adjusted upward to maintain loads that were 80% of one repetition maximum, after 1 year of training these subjects were nearing their maximum gain from the frequency and intensity employed.

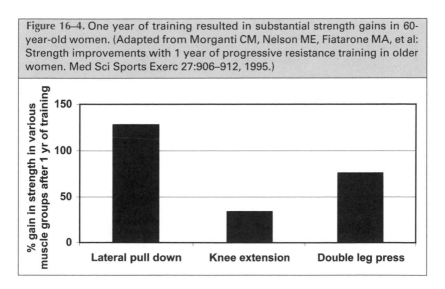

Figure 16–4. One year of training resulted in substantial strength gains in 60-year-old women. (Adapted from Morganti CM, Nelson ME, Fiatarone MA, et al: Strength improvements with 1 year of progressive resistance training in older women. Med Sci Sports Exerc 27:906–912, 1995.)

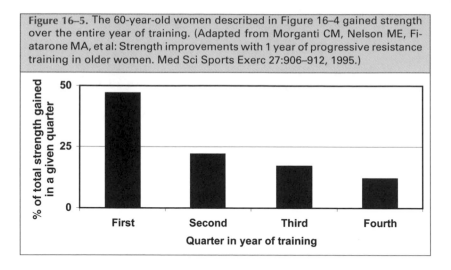

Figure 16–5. The 60-year-old women described in Figure 16–4 gained strength over the entire year of training. (Adapted from Morganti CM, Nelson ME, Fiatarone MA, et al: Strength improvements with 1 year of progressive resistance training in older women. Med Sci Sports Exerc 27:906–912, 1995.)

Even much older adults have the capacity to increase muscle strength and improve poor function (Fig. 16–6). It is well known that older individuals often do not eat enough calories and protein. In a study by Singh et al,[12] the 100% increase in muscle strength in the exercise-only group was likely due to an improved coordination of motor unit recruitment, as no significant enlargement in the diameter of individual muscle fibers occurred (Fig. 16–7). However, increases in the diameters of type II muscle fibers did occur in the group undergoing resistance training and receiving nutritional supplements.

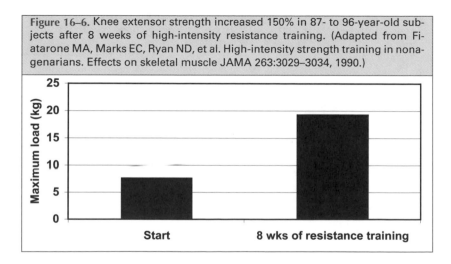

Figure 16–6. Knee extensor strength increased 150% in 87- to 96-year-old subjects after 8 weeks of high-intensity resistance training. (Adapted from Fiatarone MA, Marks EC, Ryan ND, et al. High-intensity strength training in nonagenarians. Effects on skeletal muscle JAMA 263:3029–3034, 1990.)

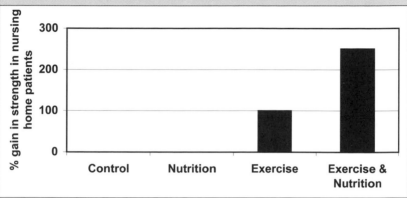

Figure 16–7. At the age of 87, nursing home patients increased their muscle strength by 250% after a combined program of resistance exercise and nutritional supplementation consisting of 360 kcal in a mix of 60% carbohydrate, 23% fat, and 17% soy-based protein. (Adapted from Singh MA, Ding W, Manfredi TJ, et al. Insulin-like growth factor-I in skeletal muscle after weight-lifting exercise in frail elders. Am J Physiol 277:E135–143, 1999.)

Resistance training also improves gait stability and balance, and leads to fewer falls in nursing home populations (Fig. 16–8). In one study, gait instability was decreased by 47% in 78-year-old individuals who underwent a 6-month, home-based strength and balance training program with encouragement to increase overall aerobic and physical activity.[13] In addition, knee extension strength increased by 42%.

Molecular mechanisms activated by loading signal skeletal muscle to hypertrophy (Fig 16–9). Future research is needed to understand how signal pathways in older individuals can be altered with resistance exercise, so as to further delay the aging process. This is important, as it is difficult to convince older individuals to undertake resistance training, and obvious and/or quick benefits would be helpful in this regard. An understanding of the molecular/cellular mechanisms producing skeletal muscle hypertrophy could improve effectiveness of resistance training.

Aerobic Capacity

Decline in aerobic capacity with aging is accompanied by decreases in muscle mass (Fig. 16–10).[14,15] Reductions in aerobic capacity are accelerated by physical inactivity (Fig 16–11).[16] Likewise, physical activity delays age-related declines in aerobic capacity. The clinical significance of a 60% higher maximal aerobic capacity is decreased mortality. In a study by Myers et al[24], a three-fold higher mortality rate occurred in the group with the lowest aerobic capacity, compared to the highest

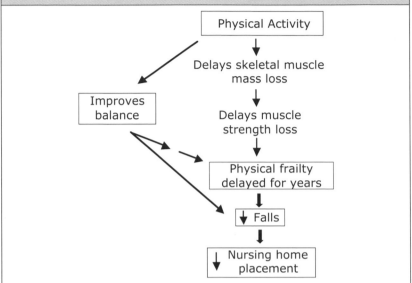

Figure 16–8. Systematically increasing muscle strength by progressive resistance training attenuates/delays age-associated decline in muscle mass, strength, and balance. This leads to improved functional capacity, ultimately delaying physical frailty.

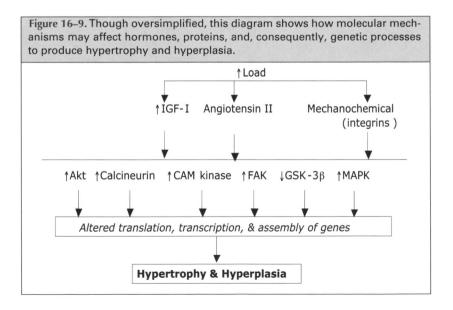

Figure 16–9. Though oversimplified, this diagram shows how molecular mechanisms may affect hormones, proteins, and, consequently, genetic processes to produce hypertrophy and hyperplasia.

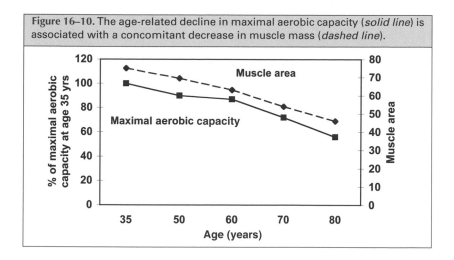

Figure 16–10. The age-related decline in maximal aerobic capacity (*solid line*) is associated with a concomitant decrease in muscle mass (*dashed line*).

aerobic capacity group. Thus, maintenance of the highest possible aerobic capacity is clinically significant in delaying death. Age-related reductions in muscle fiber size, capillaries, and mitochondria also can be delayed by aerobic training (Figs. 16–12 and 16–13).[17]

In a longitudinal study by McGuire et al, the 30-year decline in maximal aerobic capacity from a sedentary value of 50 mL O_2/kg/min at 20

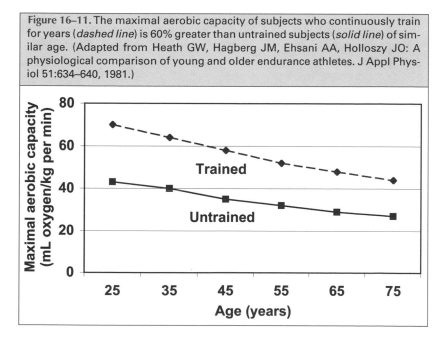

Figure 16–11. The maximal aerobic capacity of subjects who continuously train for years (*dashed line*) is 60% greater than untrained subjects (*solid line*) of similar age. (Adapted from Heath GW, Hagberg JM, Ehsani AA, Holloszy JO: A physiological comparison of young and older endurance athletes. J Appl Physiol 51:634–640, 1981.)

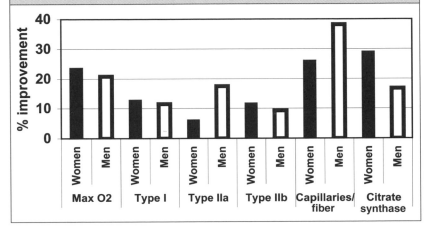

Figure 16–12. After 9–12 months of endurance training (45 min/day × 4 days/wk at 80% of maximal heart rate) in 64-year-old men and women, the improvement in whole body maximal aerobic capacity (max O₂) was accompanied by increased muscle fiber sizes (type I and IIa area), capillaries/fiber, and citrate synthase activity (which serves as index of the capacity to oxidize fuels to produce ATP) in the gastrocnemius muscle. (Adapted from Coggan AR, Spina RJ, King DS, et al: Skeletal muscle adaptations to endurance training in 60- to 70-yr-old men and women. J Appl Physiol 72:1780–1786, 1992.)

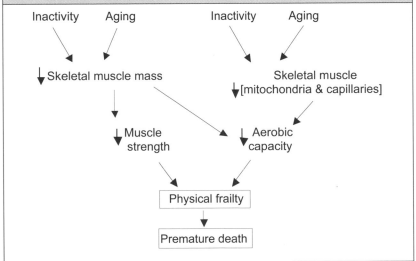

Figure 16–13. Physical inactivity speeds the onset of physical frailty and premature death during aging by causing an accelerated decrease in maximal aerobic capacity.

years of age to a sedentary value of 43 mL O_2/kg/min at 50 years of age was completely reversed to the age-20 value after 6 months of aerobic training (Fig. 16–14).[18] This recovery of the 30-year loss in maximal aerobic capacity was produced mainly by a change in peripheral oxygen extraction of the exercising skeletal muscle, because maximal cardiac output was unchanged by this training (Fig 16–15). Increased peripheral oxygen extraction during exercise was likely due to increases in the:

- Extraction of oxygen by the working skeletal muscle, possibly by increased mitochondrial and capillary densities in the trained muscle
- Efficiency of distribution of cardiac output to exercising tissues through enhanced vasoregulation and improved motor unit recruitment.

The decrease in maximal heart rate during aging was countered by an increase in maximal stroke volume and a resultant lack of change in maximal cardiac output. Current literature reports are inconclusive as to whether an improved Frank-Starling mechanism or contractility was responsible for the increased maximal stroke volume.

Aging and the Onset of Type 2 Diabetes

Prevalence of type 2 diabetes increases with aging (Fig 16–16).[19] Harris found in 1990 that by the age of 65 years, 18% of the U.S. population

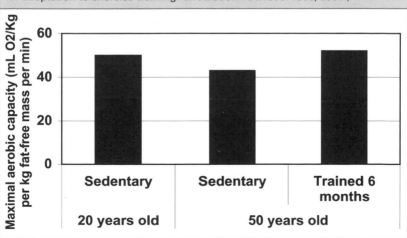

Figure 16–14. Only 6 months of aerobic training by 50-year-old subjects reversed age-related decline in maximal aerobic capacity to age-20 levels. (Adapted from McGuire DK, Levine BD, Williamson JW, et al: A 30-year follow-up of the Dallas Bedrest and Training Study—II. Effect of age on cardiovascular adaptation to exercise training. Circulation 104:1358–1366, 2001.)

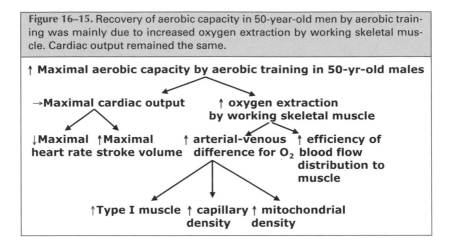

Figure 16–15. Recovery of aerobic capacity in 50-year-old men by aerobic training was mainly due to increased oxygen extraction by working skeletal muscle. Cardiac output remained the same.

has been diagnosed with diabetes. Some suggest that the increased prevalence of type 2 diabetes with aging is due to "aging genes." In fact, 91% of cases of type 2 diabetes are associated with environmental factors, and most can be prevented by a physically active lifestyle.[26]

Seals et al studied glucose tolerance in athletes and sedentary men.[20] Master's athletes (60 years old) who averaged 8 miles/day of running did *not* have the age-associated higher rise in postprandial blood glucose and insulin. Moreover, the post-meal rise in blood insulin was half that occurring in the young, untrained men. Young, untrained subjects were able to maintain normal blood glucose levels in an oral glucose toler-

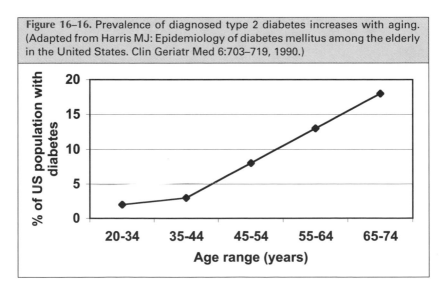

Figure 16–16. Prevalence of diagnosed type 2 diabetes increases with aging. (Adapted from Harris MJ: Epidemiology of diabetes mellitus among the elderly in the United States. Clin Geriatr Med 6:703–719, 1990.)

ance test by the pancreas compensating with a higher secretion of insulin. Increased postprandial rises in blood glucose (Fig 16–17) and insulin (Fig 16–18) in the "old, untrained, and lean" are called insulin resistance or the "prediabetic" state.

Thus, the insulin sensitivity of old Master's athletes was higher than untrained young and old subjects. Old Master's athletes had no insulin resistance, i.e., their physical activity levels were sufficient to totally prevent the so-called aging-associated increase in type 2 diabetes. The conclusion may be drawn that physical activity can delay/prevent the "age-related" onset of type 2 diabetes!

Threshold of Physical Activity Needed

Primary and Secondary Prevention

The Harvard Nurse's Health study[21] found that 30 min/day of brisk walking at 3 mph resulted in a 30% reduction in the incidence of type 2 diabetes. The weekly net caloric expenditure for a 60-kg individual walking 3.5 hrs/wk at 3 mph is approximately 840 kcal/week. (Net caloric expenditure subtracts resting metabolism to provide an estimate of calories expended by the physical activity alone.) The Washington University at St. Louis study[20] (Figs. 16–17 and 16–18) found that running 8 miles/day

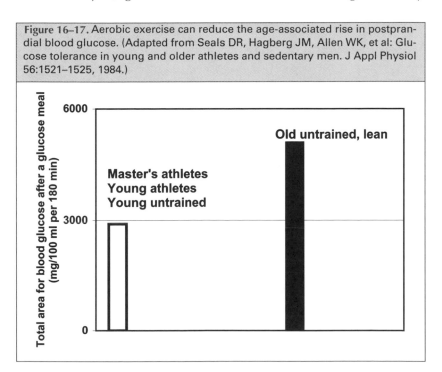

Figure 16–17. Aerobic exercise can reduce the age-associated rise in postprandial blood glucose. (Adapted from Seals DR, Hagberg JM, Allen WK, et al: Glucose tolerance in young and older athletes and sedentary men. J Appl Physiol 56:1521–1525, 1984.)

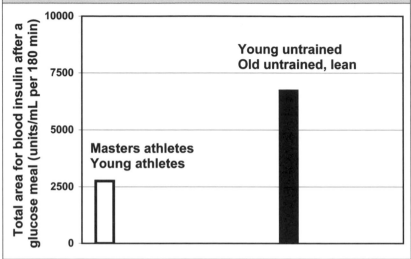

Figure 16–18. Master's athletes (60 years old) prevented the age-associated increases in postprandial blood insulin levels (i.e., insulin resistance) seen in the "old untrained lean" subjects. (Adapted from Seals DR, Hagberg JM, Allen WK, et al: Glucose tolerance in young and older athletes and sedentary men. J Appl Physiol 56:1521–1525, 1984.)

reduced type 2 diabetes by 100%. The net caloric expenditure above resting metabolism of running 8 miles/day 7 days/week is approximately 5000 kcal in a 60-kg individual. Dose-response relationships between 840 and 5000 kcal/wk to prevent 95% of type 2 diabetes by caloric expenditure alone have not yet been determined.

The recent U.S. Diabetes Prevention Program clinical trial[22] determined that 150 minutes of walking/week and other lifestyle modification reduced type 2 diabetes by 58% in subjects who were already glucose intolerant, but not yet overtly diabetic.

Hereditary Factors

The threshold of daily physical activity required to prevent type 2 diabetes is unknown. However, it is likely to be lower than running 8 miles/day. Certainly it will vary from patient to patient depending upon heredity factors. For example, the quantity of daily physical activity required to prevent type 2 diabetes is much higher for individuals with a family history of type 2 diabetes than in those without this family history (Fig. 16–19).[21] Siblings with a parental history of type 2 diabetes had at least twice the risk of themselves developing a clinical case of type 2 diabetes as compared to siblings in families without this parental history. Siblings with a parental history lowered their risk of type 2 diabetes by

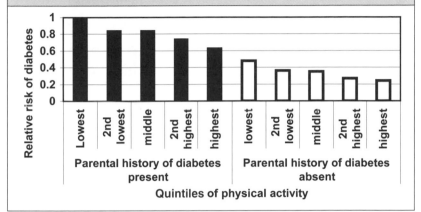

Figure 16–19. Parental history of type 2 diabetes (t2d) is a hereditary factor that increases risk. Siblings with or without a parental history of t2d reduced their risk of a clinical diagnosis by 40% by exercising in the highest quintile, but the absolute risk was twice as high in siblings with a parental history. Highest level of physical activity = an average of 34 MET-hr/wk = walking at 3 mph for 1.4 hrs/day every day or jogging at 5 mph for 36 min every day. (Adapted from Hu FB, Sigal RJ, Rich-Edwards JW, et al: Walking compared with vigorous physical activity and risk of type 2 diabetes in women: A prospective study. JAMA 282: 1433–1439, 1999.)

40% by being in the top 20% of physical activity. This is a major accomplishment as the best drug only reduced type 2 diabetes by 31%.[22]

However, even the most physically active siblings (34 MET-hrs physical activity/wk) with a parental history of type 2 diabetes had a risk level similar to that found in the most sedentary quintile of individuals with no parental history. Therefore, patients with a parental history require a prescription for more and/or perhaps higher-intensity daily physical activity.

Although those without a parental history of type 2 diabetes have a markedly lower risk than patients with this parental history, this study shows that they can still halve their risk by engaging in the highest level of physical activity—and again demonstrates an independent role for physical *in*activity in producing type 2 diabetes.

Physical Inactivity and Insulin Resistance

Insulin resistance is markedly increased by 10 days of physical inactivity in 60-year-old Master's athletes.[23] During an oral glucose tolerance test, both plasma glucose and insulin were significantly higher after 10 days of no exercise, approaching values found in type 2 diabetes, than prior to when they were exercising daily (Fig 16–20). Thus, *regular* physical activity is required to *maintain* the beneficial effects of glucose

Figure 16–20. Insulin resistance occurred when 61-year-old Master's athletes stopped exercising for 10 days. (Adapted from Rogers MA, King DS, Hagberg JM, et al. Effect of 10 days of physical inactivity on glucose tolerance in master athletes. J Appl Physiol 68:1833–1837, 1990.)

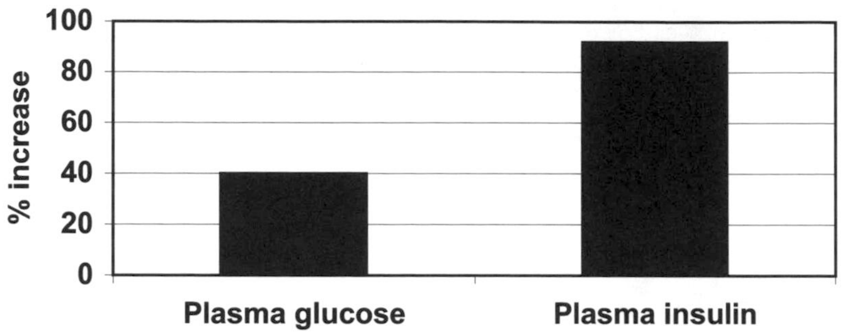

metabolism, particularly on insulin resistance, which can develop even in just a few days of inactivity.

Physical activity enhances GLUT4 protein concentration, and consequently, increases glucose uptake and insulin sensitivity in physically active skeletal muscles in both young/old men and women. Glucose uptake during maximal aerobic physical activity is directly associated with

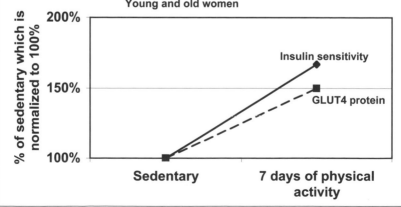

Figure 16–21. Physical activity increased GLUT4 protein in skeletal muscle and insulin sensitivity in young and old women. (Adapted from Cox JH, Cortright RN, Dohm GL, Houmard JA. Effect of aging on response to exercise training in humans: skeletal muscle GLUT-4 and insulin sensitivity. J Appl Physiol 86: 2019–2025, 1999.)

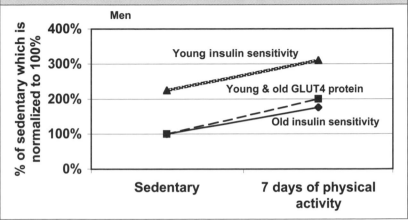

Figure 16–22. Physical activity increased GLUT4 protein in skeletal muscle and insulin sensitivity in young and old men. (Adapted from Cox JH, Cortright RN, Dohm GL, Houmard JA. Effect of aging on response to exercise training in humans: skeletal muscle GLUT-4 and insulin sensitivity. J Appl Physiol 86:2019–2025, 1999.)

the existing concentration of GLUT4 protein in skeletal muscle, which in turn is rate-limiting to the transport of glucose into muscle. Just 1 week of increased physical activity of moderate intensity enhanced both GLUT4 protein in skeletal muscle and whole-body insulin sensitivity in both young (21–22 years old) and old (57–61 years old) men and women

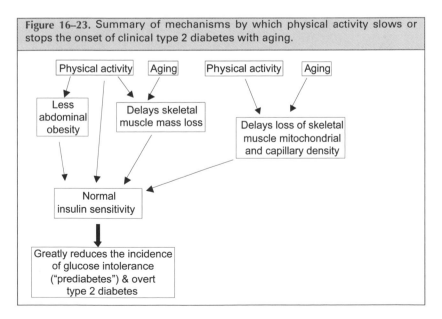

Figure 16–23. Summary of mechanisms by which physical activity slows or stops the onset of clinical type 2 diabetes with aging.

who were sedentary and undertook 7 days of cycling at 70–75% maximal aerobic capacity for 1 hour each day (Figs. 16–21 and 16–22).

Functional Capacity of Organs: Sedentary Lifestyle and Catastrophic Illness

Sedentary lifestyle is associated with reduced organ function at any given age from 20 years onward.[25] A catastrophic illness accelerates the decline in the functional capacity of organs (Fig.16–24). Recovery of organ function after a catastrophic illness in older individuals often does not occur, or is only partially successful; physical inactivity contributes to this loss. Physical activity can facilitate recovery of organ function.

The accelerated loss of functional capacity in many organ systems that is produced by a sedentary lifestyle can be primarily prevented by physical activity. Aging individuals must be encouraged to remain physically active to retain organ function. Unfortunately, periods of physical inactivity may be necessary during catastrophic illness; in such cases, loss of organ functional capacity is more rapid. If not clinically harmful

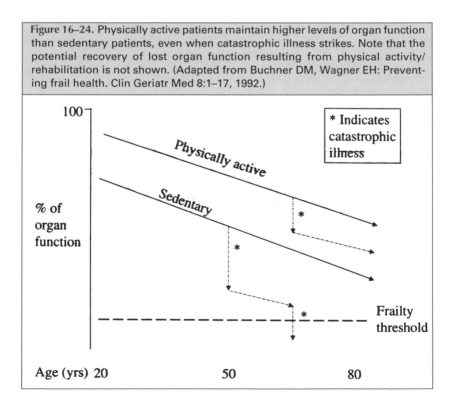

Figure 16–24. Physically active patients maintain higher levels of organ function than sedentary patients, even when catastrophic illness strikes. Note that the potential recovery of lost organ function resulting from physical activity/ rehabilitation is not shown. (Adapted from Buchner DM, Wagner EH: Preventing frail health. Clin Geriatr Med 8:1–17, 1992.)

TABLE 16–2. Loss of Organ Functional Capacity With Aging: Effects of Primary, Secondary, and Tertiary Physical Activity Preventions

Functions/Structures	Prevention Will Delay Effects of Aging		
	Primary	Secondary	Tertiary
Skeletal muscle strength	Yes	Yes	Yes
Gait/balance	Yes	Yes	Yes
Skeletal muscle fiber size	Yes	Yes	Yes
Skeletal muscle capillary density	Yes	Yes	Yes
Skeletal muscle capacity to make ATP	Yes	Yes	Yes
Maximal aerobic capacity	Yes	Yes	Yes
Frailty	Yes	Yes	Yes
Premature death due to frailty and low maximal aerobic capacity	Yes	Yes	Yes
Insulin resistance/type 2 diabetes	Yes	Yes	Yes
Skeletal muscle GLUT4	Yes	Yes	Yes
Cognitive function	Sometimes	Unknown	Unknown
Bone mass/osteoporosis	Yes	Yes	Yes

to the recovering patient, secondary prevention by physical activity is needed to minimize loss in organ function.

Upon recovery from catastrophic illness, the patient will not be able to engage in physical activity at pre-illness levels due to losses in aerobic and strength capacities. Note that failure to recover some or all of the pre-illness functional capacity initiates a vicious cycle, with reduced organ capacity leading to physical inactivity, leading to an additional loss in the functional capacity of organ systems. Consequently, special attention must be paid to prescribing physical activity and rehabilitation for these patients to prevent the downward spiral to physical frailty. Tertiary prevention of physical frailty is also possible, as demonstrated by the increased strength gains achieved by individuals in their 9th decade of life (see Figs. 16–6 and 16–7).

Suggested Reading

1. Bortz WM. Disuse and aging. JAMA 248:1203–1208, 1982.
2. Eaton SB, Strassman BI, Nesse RM, et al. Evolutionary health promotion. Prev Med 34:109–118, 2002.
3. Resnick NM: Geriatric medicine. In Fauci AS, Braunwald E, Isselbacher KJ, et al (eds): Harrison's Principles of Internal Medicine, 14th ed. New York, McGraw-Hill, 1998, p 37.
4. Spirduso WW, Cronin DL. Exercise dose-response effects on quality of life and independent living in older adults. Med Sci Sports Exerc 33: S598-S608; discussion S609–S610, 2001.
5. Keysor JJ, Jette AM. Have we oversold the benefit of late-life exercise? J Gerontol A Biol Sci Med Sci 56: M412–M423, 2001.

6. Krieger M. Ueber die atrophie der menschlichen organe bei inanition Z. angew. Anat Konstitutional 7:87–134, 1920.

7. Winick M (ed). Hunger Disease—Studies by Jewish Physicians in the Warsaw Ghetto. New York, John Wiley & Sons, 1979.

8. Diehr P, Bild DE, Harris TB, et al. Body mass index and mortality in nonsmoking older adults: The Cardiovascular Health Study. Am J Public Health 88:623–629, 1998.

9. Cornoni-Huntley JC, Harris TB, Everett DF, et al. An overview of body weight of older persons, including the impact on mortality. The National Health and Nutrition Examination Survey I—Epidemiologic Follow-up Study. J Clin Epidemiol 44:743–753, 1991.

10. Morganti CM, Nelson ME, Fiatarone MA, et al. Strength improvements with 1 year of progressive resistance training in older women. Med Sci Sports Exerc 27:906–912, 1995.

11. Fiatarone MA, Marks EC, Ryan ND, et al. High-intensity strength training in nonagenarians. Effects on skeletal muscle. JAMA 263:3029–3034, 1990.

12. Singh MA, Ding W, Manfredi TJ, et al. Insulin-like growth factor-I in skeletal muscle after weight-lifting exercise in frail elders. Am J Physiol 277:E135–143, 1999.

13. Hausdorff JM, Nelson ME, Kaliton D, et al. Etiology and modification of gait instability in older adults: a randomized controlled trial of exercise. J Appl Physiol 90: 2117–2129, 2001.

14. Fried L, Walston J. Frailty and failure to thrive. In Hazzard WR, Blass JP, Ettinger WH, et al (eds): Principles of Geriatric Medicine and Gerontology, 4th ed. New York, McGraw-Hill, 1999, pp 1387–1402.

15. Lexell J, Taylor CC, Sjostrom M. What is the cause of the ageing atrophy? Total number, size and proportion of different fiber types studied in whole vastus lateralis muscle from 15- to 83-year-old men. J Neurol Sci 84:275–294, 1988.

16. Heath GW, Hagberg JM, Ehsani AA, Holloszy JO. A physiological comparison of young and older endurance athletes. J Appl Physiol 51:634–640, 1981.

17. Coggan AR, Spina RJ, King DS, et al. Skeletal muscle adaptations to endurance training in 60- to 70-yr-old men and women. J Appl Physiol 72:1780–1786, 1992.

18. McGuire DK, Levine BD, Williamson JW, et al. A 30-year follow-up of the Dallas Bedrest and Training Study: II. Effect of age on cardiovascular adaptation to exercise training. Circulation 104:1358–1366, 2001.

19. Harris MJ. Epidemiology of diabetes mellitus among the elderly in the United States. Clin Geriatr Med 6:703–719, 1990.

20. Seals DR, Hagberg JM, Allen WK, et al. Glucose tolerance in young and older athletes and sedentary men. J Appl Physiol 56:1521–1525, 1984.

21. Hu FB, Sigal RJ, Rich-Edwards JW, et al. Walking compared with vigorous physical activity and risk of type 2 diabetes in women: A prospective study. JAMA 282:1433–1439, 1999.

22. Knowler WC, Barrett-Connor E, Fowler SE, et al; Diabetes Prevention Program Research Group. Reduction in the incidence of type 2 diabetes with lifestyle intervention or metformin. New Engl J Med 346:393–403, 2002.

23. Rogers MA, King DS, Hagberg JM, et al. Effect of 10 days of physical inactivity on glucose tolerance in master athletes. J Appl Physiol 68:1833–1837, 1990.

24. Myers J, et al. Exercise capacity and mortality among men referred for exercise testing. New Engl J Med 346:793–801, 2002.

25. Buchner DM, Wagner EH. Preventing frail health. Clin Geriatr Med 8:1–17, 1992.

26. Hu FB, et al. Diet, lifestyle, and the risk of type 2 diabetes in women. N Eng J Med 345:790–797, 2001.

Bed Rest and Spinal Cord Injury

chapter
17

"Look at a patient lying in bed.
What a pathetic picture he makes.
The blood clotting in his veins,
the lime draining from his bones,
the scybola stacking in his colon,
the flesh rotting from his sweat,
the urine leaking from his distended bladder,
and the spirit evaporating from his soul."

From Asher R: The dangers of going to bed.
Brit Med J 2:967, 1947.

In this chapter, we delineate the profound decreases in the functional capacity of organ systems induced by near-total physical inactivity. The long-term effects of no regular exercise are made clear. We also show how prescribed bed rest can be detrimental, adversely effecting the healing of many clinical conditions. For example, declines in physical activity among ICU patients represent a significant health risk.[1]

Bed Rest

Reduced Cardiovascular and Aerobic Fitness

Forced bed rest in young, healthy individuals results in a profound decrease in cardiovascular function and maximal aerobic capacity. In fact, maximal **aerobic capacity declines by 28%** after 20 days of bed rest (Fig. 17–1).[2] Remarkably, the 20-year-olds who were physically trained for 8 weeks after the 20-day bed rest completely recovered the lost aerobic capacity, so that they started aging in 1966 from a maximal aerobic capacity of 3.4 L O_2/min (data not shown).

Maximal **cardiac output declines by 26%** after 20 days of bed rest.[2] As the systemic arteriovenous difference in oxygen was unchanged during 20 days of bed rest in young, healthy men (data not shown),

245

Figure 17–1. Maximal oxygen consumption dropped more in 20 days of bed rest than it dropped due to aging from 20 to 50 years of age in the same men. The five men engaged in various levels of physical activity in the 30 years after illness (*Lifestyle 1996*) regained some capacity. (Adapted from McGuire DK, Levine BD, Williamson JW, et al. A 30-year follow-up of the Dallas Bedrest and Training Study: I. Effect of age on the cardiovascular response to exercise. Circulation 104:1350–1357, 2001.)

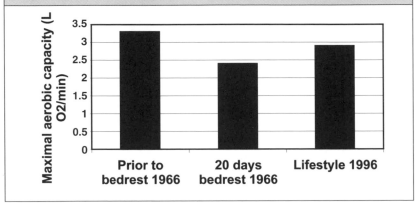

according to the Fick equation, the decrease in maximal aerobic capacity is due to a decrease in maximal cardiac output (Fig. 17–2). The loss in cardiac output was completely recovered in 20-year-olds after 8

Figure 17–2. Maximal cardiac output dropped more in 20 days of bed rest than it dropped due to aging from 20 to 50 years of age in the same men. The five men engaged in various levels of physical activity in the 30 years after illness (*Lifestyle 1996*) regained some capacity. (Adapted from McGuire DK, Levine BD, Williamson JW, et al. A 30-year follow-up of the Dallas Bedrest and Training Study: I. Effect of age on the cardiovascular response to exercise. Circulation 104:1350–1357, 2001.)

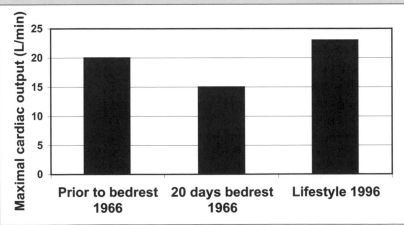

weeks of training (data not shown), and did not show any aging effect from 20 to 50 years of age.

Maximal **stroke volume declines by 29%** after 20 days of bed rest.[2] As maximal heart rate remained unchanged after 20 days of bed rest (data not shown), the decrease in maximal cardiac output after bed rest was due to the decrease in maximal stroke volume (Fig. 17–3). The loss in stroke volume was completely recovered after 8 weeks of training following 20 days of bed rest (data not shown), and did not show any aging effect from 20 to 50 years of age in men.

Other Important Changes During Bed Rest

- Increased deep vein thrombosis (DVT)—Inactivity, as brief as sitting in an airplane or car seat for 5 hours, increases the odds ratio to 4.0 for venous thromboembolic disease from a DVT.[4]
- Disuse osteoporosis—Prolonged therapeutic bed rest is a common cause of disuse osteoporosis.[5]
- Fainting—Orthostatic intolerance (due to pooling of blood in legs secondary to loss of sympathetic vasoconstriction) causes the carotid blood pressure to drop upon becoming upright after bed rest.[6]
- Decreased heart volume—Volume decreases by 11% after 20 days of bed rest in 20-year-old, healthy men.[7]
- Increased insulin resistance—Bed rest for as little as 7 days is asso-

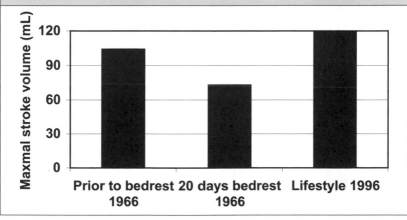

Figure 17–3. Maximal stroke volume dropped more in 20 days of bed rest than it dropped due to aging from 20 to 50 years of age in the same men. The five men engaged in various levels of physical activity in the 30 years after illness (*Lifestyle 1996*) had stroke volumes higher than their pre-bedrest levels. (Adapted from McGuire DK, Levine BD, Williamson JW, et al. A 30-year follow-up of the Dallas Bedrest and Training Study: I. Effect of age on the cardiovascular response to exercise. Circulation 104:1350–1357, 2001.)

ciated with substantial resistance to insulin's effects on glucose metabolism, and these effects occurred primarily in skeletal muscle as there was little change in insulin action on the liver.[8]

- Increased kidney stones—The propensity for the crystallization of stone-forming calcium salts was enhanced by 5 weeks of bedrest, suggesting that immobilization may confer increased risk for the formation of calcium-containing renal stones.[9]
- Increased pneumonia—Risk of pneumonia was found to be higher among bed-bound patients (54.5 vs. 13.1 per 100 discharges) in U.S. nursing homes.[10]
- Increased pressure ulcers—Nonblanchable erythema, lymphopenia, immobility, dry skin, and decreased body weight are independent and significant risk factors for pressure ulcers in hospitalized patients whose activity is limited to bed or chair.[11]
- Increased urinary tract infection—The most common complication of stroke with bed confinement of 4 days or longer was bacterial infection consisting of either pneumonia, sepsis, or urinary tract infection.[12]

Spinal Cord Injury

Decreased physical activity contributes to adverse changes resulting from spinal cord injury. Persons with spinal cord injury appear to age

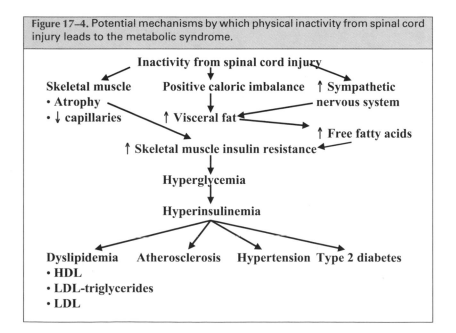

Figure 17–4. Potential mechanisms by which physical inactivity from spinal cord injury leads to the metabolic syndrome.

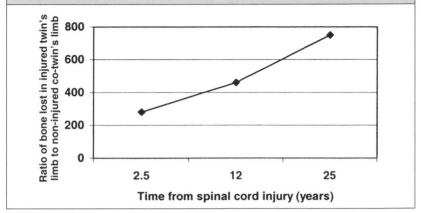

Figure 17–5. Study of physical inactivity in spinal cord injury (SCI) using co-twin control method: in this case, 8 pairs of identical male twins, one of each set with SCI. Injured twins lost a significantly greater amount of bone mass. (Data from Bauman WA, Spungen AM, Wang J, et al. Continuous loss of bone during chronic immobilization: A monozygotic twin study. Osteoporos Int 10(2):123–127, 1999.)

prematurely, in part because of secondary medical conditions, including the metabolic syndrome. (See Chapter 12 for a discussion of the metabolic syndrome.) Chronic spinal cord injury patients have an increased prevalence of dyslipidemias, atherosclerosis, hypertension, and type 2 diabetes (Fig. 17–4).[13]

Other biological processes also contribute to changes resulting from spinal cord injury[13]:

- Blunted growth hormone response to its provocative stimulator, arginine
- Decreased serum IGF-I concentrations
- Decreased serum total testosterone in male spinal cord patients
- Continued loss of leg bone mass over a protracted period of time (Fig. 17–5)[3]

Suggested Reading

1. Topp R, Ditmyer M, King K, et al. The effect of bed rest and potential of prehabilitation on patients in the intensive care unit. AACN Clin Issues 13:263–276, 2002.
2. McGuire DK, Levine BD, Williamson JW, et al. A 30-year follow-up of the Dallas Bedrest and Training Study: I. Effect of age on the cardiovascular response to exercise. Circulation 104:1350–1357, 2001.
3. Bauman WA, Spungen AM, Wang J, et al. Continuous loss of bone during chronic immobilization: A monozygotic twin study. Osteoporos Int 10(2):123–127, 1999.
4. Ferrari E, et al. Travel as a risk factor for venous thromboembolic disease: A case-control study. Chest 115:440–444, 1999.

5. Takata S, Yasui N. Disuse osteoporosis. J Med Invest 48:147–156, 2001.
6. Pavy-Le Traon A, et al. Contributory factors to orthostatic intolerance after simulated weightlessness. Clin Physiol 19:360–380, 1999.
7. Saltin B, et al. Response to exercise after bed rest and training. Circulation 38(5 Suppl) VII 1–78, 1968.
8. Stuart CA, et al. Bed-rest–induced insulin resistance occurs primarily in muscle. Metabolism 37:802–806, 1988.
9. Hwang TI, et al. Effort of prolonged bedrest on the propensity for renal stone formation. J Clin Endocrinol Metab 66:109–112, 1988.
10. Beck-Sague C, et al. Infectious diseases and mortality among U.S. nursing home residents. Am J Public Health 83:1739–1742, 1993.
11. Allman RM, et al. Pressure ulcer risk factors among hospitalized patients with activity limitation. JAMA 273:865–870, 1995.
12. Kelley RE, et al. Evaluation of kinetic therapy in the prevention of complications of prolonged bed rest secondary to stroke. Stroke 18:638–642, 1987.
13. Bauman WA, Spungen AM. Metabolic changes in persons after spinal cord injury. Phys Med Rehabil Clin North Am 11:109–140, 2000.

Pulmonary Diseases

chapter
18

Asthma

Adult Glycine-16 Allele Asthma

The epidemiology of adult-onset asthma is largely unknown. However, recent observations indicate a possible association between β_2-adrenoceptor regulation and the disorder. There is an association between high BMI and asthma, and this association is most marked among sedentary women[1]. Finally, it has been documented that those who possess the Gly16 allele have more severe adult-onset asthma symptoms (i.e., greater nocturnal symptoms, greater-than-expected frequency of steroid-dependent asthma, poorer response to therapy, and increased atopy).[1]

The significance of recognizing patients with the Gly16 allele is that this subgroup of patients is distinctly different from the subpopulation that has exercise-induced asthma, and hence forms a separate subpopulation that might be at risk of asthma associated with a *lack* of physical activity, particularly among older subjects. Remarkably, women with the Gly16 genotype were found to have no increased risk of adult-onset asthma if they were physically active (walking at a brisk pace for 1 hr/wk).[1] We speculate that physical activity may act as primary prevention of adult asthma in patients with the Gly16 allele (Fig. 18–1).

McFadden and Gilbert[4] hypothesized that at low levels of physical activity, mechanisms related to lack of deep inspirations could promote bronchospasm. More studies are needed to better document the intensity and duration of physical activity needed to produce sufficient deep inspirations to inhibit bronchospasm. Presently, very little is known about the cellular and molecular mechanisms that are affected by physical activity to produce this dramatic change. Studies on how exercise regulates gene expression of the β_2 adrenergic receptor and the interplay with the Gly16 allele are potentially fruitful avenues for further research.

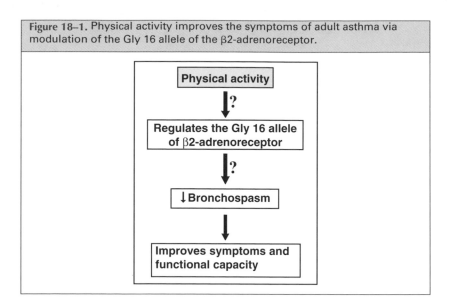

Figure 18–1. Physical activity improves the symptoms of adult asthma via modulation of the Gly 16 allele of the β2-adrenoreceptor.

Exercise-Associated Asthma

This is a condition in which vigorous physical activity triggers acute airway narrowing in people with heightened airway reactivity.[4] A high prevalence of asthma and airway hyperresponsiveness has been reported in the athlete population. Factors potentially predisposing athletes to these conditions have not been clearly identified, although relevant preventive and therapeutic measures have been suggested. Habitual physical activity has been shown to reduce the likelihood of provoking exercise-induced asthma.[5]

Chronic Obstructive Pulmonary Disease

There is no evidence suggesting that physical *in*activity increases the occurrence of COPD; therefore, primary and secondary prevention by physical activity are not applicable. It is known, however, that patients with COPD have significantly reduced levels of physical activity and often avoid exertion because of the fear of dyspnea. Deconditioning from disuse is believed to be a major contributing factor in the skeletal muscle dysfunction that is observed in patients with COPD. They have weak skeletal muscles with reduced mitochondrial density. Peripheral muscle dysfunction is a common systemic complication of moderate to severe COPD and may contribute to disability, handicap, and premature mortality.

As for tertiary prevention, endurance exercise training has been conclusively demonstrated to improve exercise tolerance in COPD.[2] In contrast to the lung impairment, which is largely irreversible, peripheral muscle

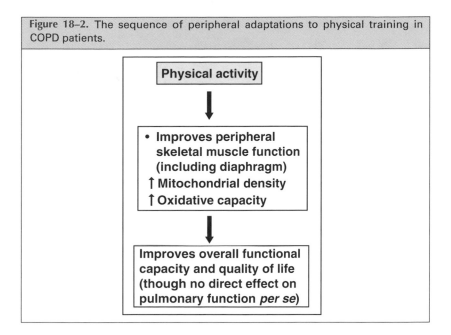

Figure 18–2. The sequence of peripheral adaptations to physical training in COPD patients.

Physical activity

- Improves peripheral skeletal muscle function (including diaphragm)
↑ Mitochondrial density
↑ Oxidative capacity

Improves overall functional capacity and quality of life (though no direct effect on pulmonary function *per se*)

dysfunction is potentially remediable with exercise training. Pulmonary rehabilitation is now established as effective treatment to improve the quality of life for patients with COPD, and it is clear that, if exercised at appropriate intensities, COPD patients show improved metabolic adaptations to training.[3] Respiratory rehabilitation, including lower limb exercise training, is now recommended as part of the management for COPD patients, because it has been consistently shown that this relieves dyspnea and improves health-related quality of life.

Currently, the cellular mechanisms behind exercise effects on pulmonary physiology of patients with COPD are unknown (Fig. 18–2).

Suggested Reading

1. Barr RG, Cooper DM, Speizer FE, et al. Beta(2)-adrenoceptor polymorphism and body mass index are associated with adult-onset asthma in sedentary but not active women. Chest 120:1474–1479, 2001.
2. Casaburi R. Skeletal muscle dysfunction in chronic obstructive pulmonary disease. Med Sci Sports Exerc 33(7 Suppl):S662–670, 2001.
3. Steiner MC, Morgan MD. Enhancing physical performance in chronic obstructive pulmonary disease. Thorax 56: 73–77, 2001.
4. McFadden ER Jr, Gilbert IA. Exercise-induced asthma. N Engl J Med 330: 1362–1367, 1994.
5. Ram FS, Robinson SM, Black PN. Physical training for asthma. Cochrane Database Syst Rev 2000; (2):CD001116.

Inflammation/ Immune System Dysfunction

HOT TOPICS

Infection

Prolonged, heavy exertion has an adverse effect on many components of the immune system. Resultant immune changes have been noted in the skin, upper respiratory tract mucosal tissue, lung, blood, and muscle. Nieman speculates that during the immediate period (3–72 hrs) after the prolonged, heavy exercise, an "open window" of impaired immunity exists during which viruses and bacteria may gain a foothold, increasing the risk of subclinical and clinical infection.[4] The infection risk may be amplified when other factors related to immune function are present, including exposure to novel pathogens during travel on an airplane, lack of sleep, severe mental stress, malnutrition, or weight loss (Fig. 19–1).

Blood Markers of Inflammation

Since elevated levels of C-reactive protein and other markers of inflammation are important predictors of increased coronary heart disease risk, it has been hypothesized that reducing inflammation could in fact lower the risk of coronary heart disease (Fig. 19–2).

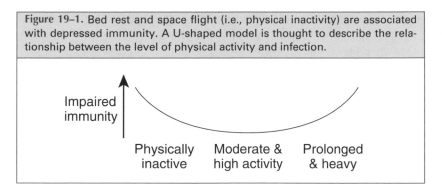

Figure 19–1. Bed rest and space flight (i.e., physical inactivity) are associated with depressed immunity. A U-shaped model is thought to describe the relationship between the level of physical activity and infection.

Impaired immunity

Physically inactive   Moderate & high activity   Prolonged & heavy

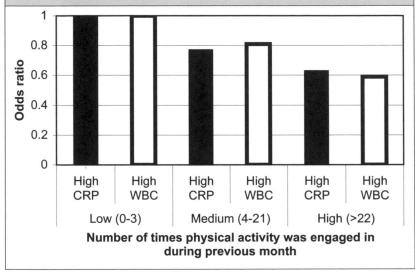

Figure 19-2. Higher frequencies of physical activity were associated with significantly lower odds of having elevated C-reactive protein (CRP) and white blood cells (WBC) in 3600 apparently healthy U.S. men and women who were ≥ 40 years old. (Adapted from Abramson JL, Vaccarino V: Relationship between physical activity and inflammation among apparently healthy middle-aged and older U.S. adults. Arch Intern Med 162:1286–1292, 2002.)

Cancer

Woods et al[2] suggested the hypothesis underlying Figure 19–1, which states that *moderate-intensity* physical activity will enhance immune system function, and thereby reduce the susceptibility to cancer. In contrast, the numbers and function of cells mediating cytotoxic activity against virus-infected cells are suppressed after repeated bouts of exhaustive exercise, and this may lead to decreased immune system function and elevated susceptibility to cancer. Physical activity of moderate intensity improves a number of immune system parameters that may be important in cancer defense.[5] However, many questions remain unanswered regarding whether moderate physical activity reduces cancer risk directly through immune system modulation, or via other indirect means.

Immune System Mechanisms

The mechanisms underlying exercise-associated immune changes are multifactorial and include multiple neuroendocrine factors. This subject is beyond the scope of this book. Hence, the reader is referred to an excellent comprehensive review by Pedersen and Hoffman-Goetz.[3] Currently, little information is available describing biochemical mechanisms by which the immune system senses the difference between moderate-intensity exercise and no exercise.

Suggested Reading

1. Abramson JL, Vaccarino V. Relationship between physical activity and inflammation among apparently healthy middle-aged and older U.S. adults. Arch Intern Med 162: 1286–1292, 2002.
2. Woods JA, Davis JM, Smith JA, Nieman DC. Exercise and cellular innate immune function. Med Sci Sports Exerc 31(1):57–66, 1999.
3. Pedersen BK, Hoffman-Goetz L. Exercise and the immune system: regulation, integration, and adaptation. Physiol Rev 80:1055–1081, 2000.
4. Nieman DC. Is infection risk linked to exercise workload? Med Sci Sports Exerc 32 (7 Suppl):5406–5411, 2000.
5. Shephard RJ, Shek PN. Associations between physical activity and susceptibility to cancer: Possible mechanisms. Sports Med 26(5):293–315, 1998.

Neurological Disorders

Cognitive Dysfunction/Alzheimer's/Dementia

Epidemiology

Roughly 4 million Americans currently have Alzheimer's disease, and this number is projected to increase to 16–19 million by 2050 (National Institute on Aging and U.S. Census Bureau).

In a large-scale, prospective cohort study by Laurin et al, high levels of physical activity in ≥ 65-year-old women were associated with reduced risks of 42%, 50%, and 37% for cognitive impairment, Alzheimer's disease, and dementia of any type, respectively.[1] A significant dose-response relationship showed decreasing risk with increasing levels of physical activity. Men did not show this effect in the same study, and the investigators speculated that the number of male subjects could have been too small. Laurin et al hypothesized that the neuroprotection might have been attained by sustaining cerebral blood flow; by limiting increases in resting blood pressures, lowering lipid levels, inhibiting platelet aggregability, and enhancing cerebral metabolic demands; by improving cerebral nutrient supply and angiogenesis; or by a combination of the above. These hypotheses have yet to be proven.

Sedentary lifestyle may be a risk factor in neurodegenerative diseases because it is associated with higher risk of stroke and is more pronounced in the elderly.[3] Studies have found that physical activity either delays loss of, or has no effect on, cognitive function in elderly subjects.[2] However, no studies have reported an accelerated loss of cognitive function with physical activity.

Lindsay et al[2] have suggested that regular physical activity could represent a novel and safe preventive strategy against Alzheimer's disease and many other conditions, and it should be examined further. Interestingly, among patients with COPD, acute exercise was associated with improved performance on the verbal fluency test, a measure of verbal processing.[12]

Intermediate Mechanisms

Several animal studies indicate a beneficial effect of exercise on the **central nervous system** (CNS), and are described briefly here.

- Aged sedentary rats had 11% fewer Purkinje cells and 9% smaller Purkinje cell soma volumes than aged rats who exercised.[13] Indeed, aged rats that exercised had the same number of Purkinje cells as young rats, thereby suggesting that the degree of age-associated degenerative changes in parts of the CNS are dependent on earlier lifestyle and health habits, and may be prevented or delayed by physical exercise.
- Physical activity in rats produced 2- to 12-fold enhancements in spatial learning performance on both the Morris and place learning-set probe trials, respectively.[14]
- Physical activity also attenuated motor deficits and impeded age-related neuronal loss.[13]
- Physical activity increased the discharge frequency of pyramidal cells and interneurons as long as the animal ran continuously on the wheel. Furthermore, the discharge frequency of pyramidal cells and interneurons increased with increasing running velocity, even though the frequency of hippocampal theta waves remained constant.[15]

Cellular Mechanisms

Neuroprotection. Carro et al[3] found that physical activity reduced the vulnerability to brain damage in models of neuronal injury involving different types of etiopathogenic mechanisms relevant to human disease (Fig 20–1). Physical *in*activity may increase the susceptibility to neurodegenerative processes attributable to insufficient brain uptake of serum IGF-I.

Neurogenesis. Voluntary running on wheels by mice increased neural cell proliferation and survival by producing a net neurogenesis in the dentate gyrus of the hippocampus, which was associated with a better learning performance.[4] By comparison, physical inactivity is related to a lower level of learning performance and fewer brain cells in rats.

Neurotransmitters. Endurance-trained, adult rats showed a reduction in high-affinity choline uptake and an increase in muscarinic quinuclidinylbenzilate binding in the hippocampus, compared with their age-matched sedentary controls.[5] It is possible, then, that physical inactivity leads to a reversal of these mechanisms.

Neurotrophic factors. Voluntary running was associated with an increase in the level of the activated transcription factor, CREB phosphorylation at Ser-133, in the rat hippocampus for at least 1 week, but not after 1 month. Phosphorylated MAPK (both p42 and p44) was increased for at least 1 month.[6] Shen et al[6] interpreted these observations to be consistent

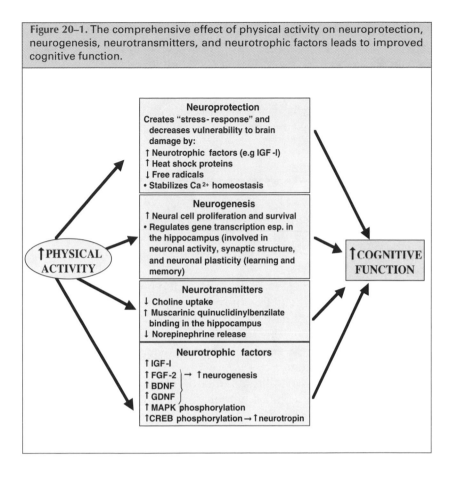

Figure 20–1. The comprehensive effect of physical activity on neuroprotection, neurogenesis, neurotransmitters, and neurotrophic factors leads to improved cognitive function.

with the view that the relatively long-lasting activation of these signaling molecules modulates the regulation of neurotropin genes, and thus contributes to the beneficial effects of physical exercise on brain function.

Voluntary running exercise has been shown to increase the number of new neurons in the adult hippocampus.[4] Because peripheral administration of IGF-I also resulted in increases in the number of new neurons in the hippocampus of hypophysectomized rats, Trejo et al[7] speculated that circulating IGF-I might be mediating the stimulatory effects of exercise on the number of new hippocampal neurons in normal adult rats. They observed a complete inhibition of the exercise-induced increase in the number of new neurons in the hippocampus when IGF-I antiserum was infused into rats undergoing exercise training. They interpreted this finding to be a result of the antibody blocking the entrance of circulating IGF-I into the brain.

Sedentary animals showed reduced brain uptake of serum IGF-I compared with exercising animals.[3] Neurons accumulating IGF-I exhibit an enhanced spontaneous firing and a protracted increase in sensitivity to afferent stimulation.

Finally, the expression of fibroblast growth factor-2, brain-derived neurotrophic factor, and glial cell-derived neurotrophic factor in the brain was decreased in sedentary rats, as compared to physically active rats.[4]

Parkinson's Disease

Clinical Studies

Physical activity is probably the most important adjunctive therapy for Parkinson's disease (Fig. 20–2), and can be beneficial for patients in all stages of the disease.[8,9] Three key benefits of physical activity in Parkinson's disease patients are:

1. Significant improvement in preventing the impairment in mobility and functional activity that results as a consequence of the major symptoms of the disease (i.e., bradykinesia, tremor, postural instability, and rigidity). This functional improvement is noted in all stages of the disease, even though physical activity has no direct effect on the symptoms *per se.*
2. Positive effects on mobility and mood. A regular and focused physical activity that includes aerobic, stretching, and strengthening activities—primarily aimed at improving flexibility and strength, rather than adding bulk—is necessary.
3. Energy preservation for the most important activities of the day. Physical activity counteracts fatigue, a major symptom of the disease.

Mechanisms

Tillerson et al[10] showed a remarkable attenuation of the loss in striatal dopaminergic neurons with increasing levels of physical activity. However, the precise biochemical mechanisms underlying this process are currently unknown.

Stroke

The role of the cardiovascular system in initiating stroke was presented in Chapter 13. Here, only the rehabilitative aspects of stroke are discussed.

In one study, a greater intensity of leg rehabilitation improved functional recovery and health-related functional status in stroke patients.[16] Moreover, supported treadmill ambulation training improved work capacity.

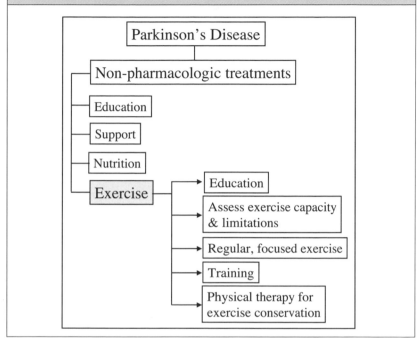

Figure 20–2. Emerging clinical data suggest that physical activity increasingly forms a core feature in the management of Parkinson's disease. (Adapted from Olanow CW, Watts RL, Koller WC. An algorithm (decision tree) for the management of Parkinson's disease: Treatment guidelines. Neurology 56(11 Suppl 5): S1–S88, 2001.)

Locomotor activity in animals before global cerebral ischemia was highly efficient in protecting the brain, as demonstrated by enhanced survival and a reduction of tissue damage, compared to sedentary animals.[17]

Liepert et al found that a use-dependent cortical plasticity occurs as a result of the increased use of body parts in behaviorally relevant tasks.[11] Constraint-induced movement therapy was applied to chronic stroke patients by restricting the usage of the nonparetic arm, and by forcing usage of the affected, paretic arm (via physical therapy for 6 hrs/day) for 8 days of the 12-day treatment course. The outcome was that the cortical representation area of the affected hand muscle in the affected hemisphere was significantly enlarged post-treatment, corresponding to a greatly improved motor performance of the affected, paretic limb.

Suggested Reading

1. Laurin D, Verreault R, Lindsay J, et al. Physical activity and risk of cognitive impairment and dementia in elderly persons. Arch Neurol 58:498–504, 2001.

2. Lindsay J, Laurin D, Verreault R, et al. Risk factors for Alzheimer's disease: A prospective analysis from the Canadian Study of Health and Aging. Am J Epidemiol 156:445–453, 2002.
3. Carro E, Trejo JL, Busiguina S, Torres-Aleman I. Circulating insulin-like growth factor I mediates the protective effects of physical exercise against brain insults of different etiology and anatomy. J Neurosci 21: 5678–5684, 2001.
4. van Praag H, Kempermann G, Gage FH. Neural consequences of environmental enrichment. Nat Rev Neurosci 1: 191–198, 2000.
5. Fordyce DE, Farrar RP. Effect of physical activity on hippocampal high affinity choline uptake and muscarinic binding: A comparison between young and old F344 rats. Brain Res 541: 57–62, 1991.
6. Shen H, Tong L, Balazs R, Cotman CW. Physical activity elicits sustained activation of the cyclic AMP response element-binding protein and mitogen-activated protein kinase in the rat hippocampus. Neuroscience 107: 219–229, 2001.
7. Trejo JL, Carro E, Torres-Aleman I. Circulating insulin-like growth factor I mediates exercise-induced increases in the number of new neurons in the adult hippocampus. J Neurosci 21: 1628–1634, 2001.
8. Koller WC. Treatment of early Parkinson's disease. Neurology 58(4 Suppl 1):S79–86, 2002.
9. Olanow CW, Watts RL, Koller WC. An algorithm (decision tree) for the management of Parkinson's disease: Treatment guidelines. Neurology 56(11 Suppl 5):S1–S88, 2001.
10. Tillerson JL, Cohen AD, Philhower J, et al. Forced limb-use effects on the behavioral and neurochemical effects of 6-hydroxydopamine. J Neurosci. 21:4427–4435, 2001.
11. Liepert J, Bauder H, Wolfgang HR, et al. Treatment-induced cortical reorganization after stroke in humans. Stroke 31:1210–1216, 2000.
12. Emery CF, Honn VJ, Frid DJ, et al. Acute effects of exercise on cognition in patients with chronic obstructive pulmonary disease. Am J Respir Crit Care Med 164:1624–1627, 2001.
13. Larsen JO, Skalicky M, Viidik A. Does long-term physical exercise counteract age-related purkinje cell loss? A stereological study of rat cerebellum. J Comp Neurol 428:213–222, 2000.
14. Fordyce DE, Wehner JM. Physical activity enhances spatial learning performance with an associated alteration in hippocampal protein kinase c activity in C57BL/6 and DBA/2 mice. Brain Res 619:111–119, 1993.
15. Czurko A, Mirase H, Csicsvari J, Buzsaki G. Sustained activation of hippocampal pyramidal cells by "space clamping" in a running wheel. Eur J Neurosci 11:344–352, 1999.
16. Kwakkel G, Wagenaar RC, Twisk JW, et al. Intensity of leg and arm training after primary middle-cerebral artery stroke: A randomized trial. Lancet 354(9174):191–196, 1999.
17. Stummer W, Weber K, Tranmer B, et al. Reduced mortality and brain damage after locomotor activity in gerbil forebrain ischemia. Stroke 25(9):1862–1869, 1994.

Musculoskeletal Disorders

chapter

21

Arthritis

Osteoarthritis

Osteoarthritis is predominantly characterized by erosion of the articular cartilage due to either primary or secondary trauma (as seen with repeated use), mostly on weight-bearing joints. A consensus report states that there is no evidence for a preventive effect of physical activity on osteoarthritis in weight-bearing joints.[5] Also, there is no evidence that inactivity of a joint alone directly produces osteoarthritis. However, physical inactivity is often associated with obesity, and obesity increases the risk of osteoarthritis. Moreover, individuals with osteoarthritis who are inactive for prolonged periods of time are likely to have poor aerobic capacity and therefore are at increased risk for cardiovascular disease and other inactivity-related conditions.

Epidemiologic studies have demonstrated that participation in certain competitive sports demanding high-intensity, acute, direct joint impact as a result of contact with other participants, playing surfaces, or equipment increases the risk for osteoarthritis.[1] Repetitive joint impact and torsional loading (twisting) also appear to be associated with joint degeneration, as seen in the elbows of baseball pitchers and the knees of soccer players. Note, however, that those who engage in moderate-intensity physical activity are at zero to low risk of osteoarthritis.

The fact that low-intensity running has perhaps no association with osteoarthritis, whereas soccer does, illustrates the concept that appropriate physical activities should be selected for reduced risk of chronic health conditions. Not all types of exercise are associated with development of osteoarthritis.

It is well recognized that patients with osteoarthritis of the knee develop quadriceps muscle weakness, which is often attributed to physical inactivity and is presumed to develop because the patient minimizes use of the painful limb.[1] Evidence is also growing that deconditioned muscle,

265

inadequate motion, and periarticular stiffness may contribute to signs and symptoms of osteoarthritis.[1,2]

Exercise is integral in reducing impairment, improving function, and preventing disability in osteoarthritic patients.[2] Some of the physical activity benefits accruing in patients with osteoarthritis are: flexibility, muscular conditioning, and cardiovascular and general health. Both therapeutic and recreational physical activity (especially that of moderate intensity and duration) is an effective therapy for the successful management of osteoarthritis.

Rheumatoid Arthritis

Rheumatoid arthritis is a chronic disease of the joints, usually symmetric polyarthritis, marked by inflammatory changes in the synovial membranes and articular structures and by atrophy and rarefaction of the bones. It is generally more common in females than males. There is no evidence that exercise prevents rheumatoid arthritis.

Previously, the cornerstone of treatment of active rheumatoid arthritis was bed rest, and patients were restrained from active physical exercise based upon the presumption of its detrimental effect on disease activity and joint erosiveness. However, inactivity as a treatment for rheumatoid arthritis is now *contraindicated,* based on several studies that uniformly show that physical therapy and moderate-intensity exercise not only reduce hand pain, stiffness, and joint tenderness, but also improve activity-of-daily-living scores.[3]

The intensity of the exercise should be well matched with the disease activity to best meet each person's needs, taking into account the severity of the arthritis, the patient's other medical problems, and the patient's individual lifestyle and preferences. Physical *in*activity results in muscle atrophy and bone loss, even in healthy individuals. Exercise in patients with rheumatoid arthritis appears to minimize loss in muscle strength, but not the loss in bone density.[4] The mechanisms by which physical activity reduces pain, stiffness, and joint tenderness in patients with rheumatoid arthritis are not well understood.

For information on osteoporosis, please refer to Chapters 16 and 23. For information on physical frailty, please refer to Chapter 16.

Suggested Reading

1. Felson DT, Lawrence RC, Dieppe PA, et al. Osteoarthritis: New insights. Part 1: The disease and its risk factors. Ann Intern Med 133: 635–646, 2000.
2. Minor MA. Exercise in the treatment of osteoarthritis. Rheum Dis Clin North Am 25: 397–415, 1999.
3. Buljina AI, Taljanovic MS, Avdic DM, Hunter TB. Physical and exercise therapy for treatment of the rheumatoid hand. Arthritis Rheum 45: 392–397, 2001.

4. Hakkinen A, Sokka T, Kotaniemi A, Hannonen P. A randomized two-year study of the effects of dynamic strength training on muscle strength, disease activity, functional capacity, and bone mineral density in early rheumatoid arthritis. Arthritis Rheum 44: 515–522, 2001.
5. Kesaniemi YA, Danforth E Jr, Jensen MD, et al. Dose-response issues concerning physical activity and health: Evidence-based symposium. Med Sci Sports Exerc 33:5351–5358, 2001.

Gastroesophageal Reflux Disease

chapter
22

Gastroesophageal reflux disease is an important cause of morbidity in the U.S.[1] Clark et al[2] initially reported that acute vigorous physical activity (running) can induce gastrointestinal reflux in normal healthy subjects. Moreover, postprandial running exercises further exacerbated reflux symptoms (secondary to disorganized esophageal motility) and correlates with exercise intensity.[3] However, in a survey of runners and age, gender-matched sedentary subjects, Sullivan et al[4] reported that upper gastrointestinal symptoms of heartburn, vomiting, and bloating were rare in runners during training, but became more common when these same runners stopped training, and was similar in frequency to the sedentary control subjects. Indeed the findings from the National Health and Nutritional Examination Survey, which followed 12,349 partici-

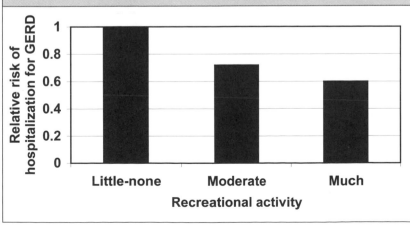

Figure 22–1. Age-adjusted risk for hospitalization with GERD is decreased with increases in recreational activity levels. (Data from Ruhl CE, Everhart JE: Overweight, but not high dietary fat intake, increases risk of gastroesophageal reflux disease hospitalization: The NHANES I Epidemiologic Follow-up Study. First National Health and Nutrition Examination Survey. Ann Epidemiol 9:424–435, 1999.)

pants over a 20-year period, showed that individuals who have been physically active over a long period of time have a lower risk of gastroesophageal reflux disease than do sedentary persons (Fig. 22-1).

Suggested Reading

1. Ruhl CE, Everhart JE. Overweight, but not high dietary fat intake, increases risk of gastroesophageal reflux disease hospitalization: The NHANES I Epidemiologic Follow-up Study. First National Health and Nutrition Examination Survey. Ann Epidemiol 9:424–435, 1999.
2. Clark CS, Kraus BB, Sinclair J, Castell DO. Gastroesophageal reflux induced by exercise in healthy volunteers. JAMA 261(24):3599–3601, 1989.
3. Choi SC, Yoo KH, Kim TH, et al. Effect of graded running on esophageal motility and gastroesophageal reflux in fed volunteers. J Korean Med Sci 16(2):183–187, 2001.
4. Sullivan SN, Wing C, Meidenheim P. Does running cause gastrointestinal symptoms? A survey of 93 randomly selected runners compared with controls. NZ Med J 107 (984):328–331, 1994.

Women's Health

chapter
23

Breast Cancer

Epidemiology

Twenty-three of 35 studies conducted to date show a decreased risk in breast cancer in women who are physically active.[1] The greatest risk reductions occurred in those going from a sedentary lifestyle to moderate-intensity physical activity.

Observations from 26 of 41 studies including 108,000 breast cancer cases demonstrated that both occupational physical activity and leisure-time physical activity were associated with a 30% reduction in breast cancer risk in pre-, peri-, and postmenopausal women, with a graded dose-response relationship reported in 16 of 28 studies.[2] Differences in study outcomes could be due to a variable association between physical activity and breast cancer across the lifespan and hormonal status of the women.

Lee et al[3] analyzed nearly 40,000 women and concluded that physical inactivity may increase the risk of all breast cancer only in post-menopausal women. Postmenopausal women who walked at least 2 miles per day experienced a risk reduction of 33% compared with those walking only a quarter mile per day. This relationship did *not* hold in post-menopausal women with breast cancers positive for estrogen or progesterone receptors. But in a specific subcategory of women, a 33% reduction in breast cancer was found.

Breast cancer has multiple causes. It is interesting to consider that if physical *in*activity accentuates only one of these causes, study outcomes will differ. This may explain the varying results often obtained.

Biochemical/Cellular Mechanisms

Some aspects of sex and metabolic hormone patterns throughout life are likely responsible for a large number of breast cancer occurrences. As physical activity modulates these sex and metabolic hormone patterns,[4] it is possible that physical activity–induced adaptations play some role in the

271

breast cancer-physical activity association (Fig 23–1). The underlying bio-chemical/cellular processes by which physical activity may alter mechanisms and decrease the risk of breast cancer are largely unknown.

Osteoporosis

Epidemiology

Osteoporosis is an age-related reduction in bone mass and density that ultimately increases a person's susceptibility to fractures. Hip fractures were associated with a 20% increase in overall mortality and 300,000 hospital admissions in 1995.[10] Moreover, health costs necessary to manage fractures that year exceeded $13.8 billion.[10]

Bone loss is continual with aging in the sedentary individual (Fig. 23–2). Women reach frailty before men because they start with smaller bones at the age of 30 years, and they lose the estrogen-promotion of bone accretion at menopause. The percentage of individuals over 65 years of age having osteopenia (reduced bone density, Fig. 23–3) and osteoporosis (more severely reduced bone density, Fig. 23–4) is very high. Osteoporosis is especially pronounced in women: 50% of women older than 85 have osteoporosis, compared to only ~10% of men the same age. This disorder does develop in men, but at a much delayed rate.

Epidemiological data indicates that bed rest markedly accelerates bone loss. Significant quantities of bone mineral were lost in healthy sub-

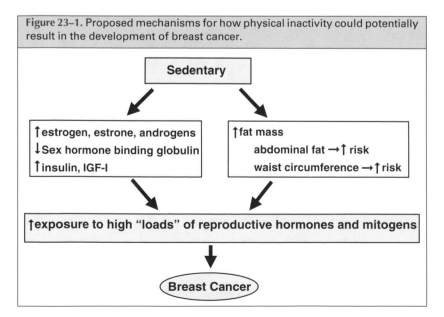

Figure 23–1. Proposed mechanisms for how physical inactivity could potentially result in the development of breast cancer.

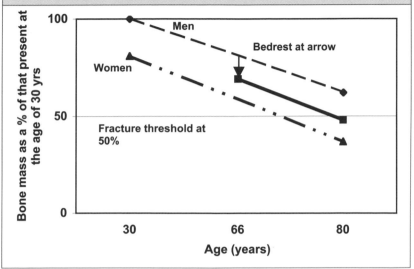

Figure 23–2. Bone mass peaks in young adult men and women, and declines thereafter, reaching a "fracture threshold" at an earlier age in women than men. Even a relatively brief period of immobility (*arrow, solid line*) results in a premature arrival at this threshold. (Data from Katz MS: Geriatrics grand rounds: Eve's rib, or a revisionist view of osteoporosis in men. J Gerontol A Biol Sci Med Sci 55:M560–M569, 2000.)

jects after 17 weeks of bed rest (Fig. 23–5).[6] The amount of loss seems to be greatest caudally. Immobilized patients can lose up to 40% of their original bone mineral density in 1 year, whereas standing upright for as little as 30 minutes per day prevents this bone loss.

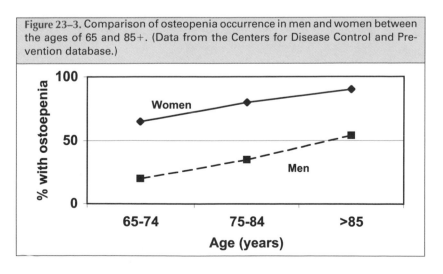

Figure 23–3. Comparison of osteopenia occurrence in men and women between the ages of 65 and 85+. (Data from the Centers for Disease Control and Prevention database.)

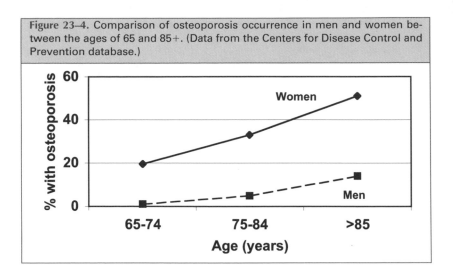

Figure 23–4. Comparison of osteoporosis occurrence in men and women between the ages of 65 and 85+. (Data from the Centers for Disease Control and Prevention database.)

Primary Prevention of Osteoporosis

Current evidence indicates that three environmental factors accelerate bone loss:
- Physical inactivity
- Insufficient nutrient and calcium intake
- Reduced female reproductive hormones.

Physical inactivity speeds the onset of osteoporosis with aging (Fig 23–6). Broken hips in elderly individuals is associated with increased mortality.

Figure 23–5. Amount of bone loss in various body areas after 17 weeks of bed rest. (Data from Leblanc AD, Schneider VS, Evans HJ, et al: Bone mineral loss and recovery after 17 weeks of bed rest. J Bone Miner Res 5:843–850, 1990.)

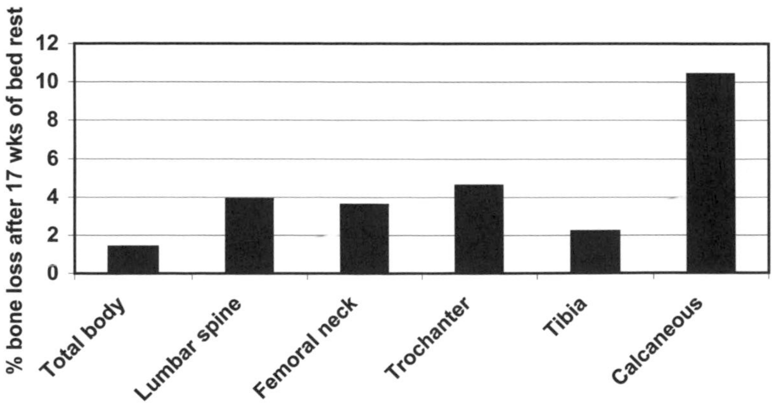

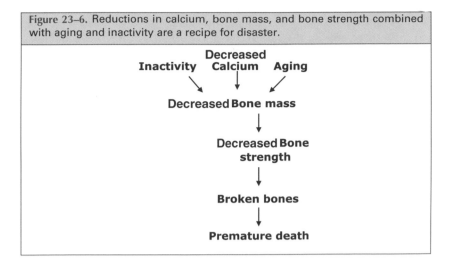

Figure 23–6. Reductions in calcium, bone mass, and bone strength combined with aging and inactivity are a recipe for disaster.

The results from the National Osteoporosis Risk Assessment (NORA) indicate that people who have a history of regular exercise have a significantly reduced risk of developing osteoporosis.[7] Appropriate physical activity, such as a chronic loading type, delays osteoporosis and prevents loss of bone mass (Fig. 23–7).[8]

Low bone mineral density (BMD) is the single best predictor of fracture risk. The formation of new bone occurs through the sensation of

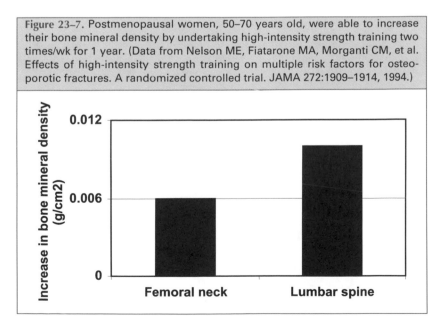

Figure 23–7. Postmenopausal women, 50–70 years old, were able to increase their bone mineral density by undertaking high-intensity strength training two times/wk for 1 year. (Data from Nelson ME, Fiatarone MA, Morganti CM, et al. Effects of high-intensity strength training on multiple risk factors for osteoporotic fractures. A randomized controlled trial. JAMA 272:1909–1914, 1994.)

strain imposed via an unaccustomed direction or distribution. In fact, exercise intervention programs have found increases of 1–5% in BMD in young populations. In the elderly, load-bearing exercise interventions can increase BMD by 5–8%. Although not all studies indicate that exercise programs can increase BMD, most do suggest that load-bearing activities such as standing, walking, and resistance training can reduce the rate of bone loss, and thereby maintain bone mass during aging.

As bone mass peaks around the age of 20, primary prevention means that increases in bone mass must be emphasized in childhood and adolescence, i.e., factors detrimental to the addition of bone mass in development should be avoided. After the second decade of life, emphasis needs to be placed on maintaining existing bone mass.

Secondary Prevention of Osteoporosis

Though bed rest significantly depletes bone mineral, recovery is possible (albeit incomplete) with reambulation and load bearing. Bone mineral recovered only partially after 17 weeks of bed rest in healthy 35-year-old male subjects who reambulated for 6 months (Fig. 23–8).[6] The trochanter only regained 26% of its lost bone mineral, meaning that it had 3.4% less bone mineral than prior to the 17 weeks of bed rest. Similar results were noted for the femoral neck and lumbar spine, which recovered 0% and 16%, respectively. This represents a deficit of 3.6% and 3.2 % of bone mineral even after 6 months of reambulation.

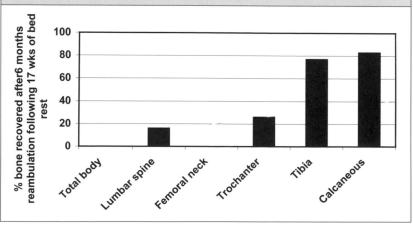

Figure 23–8. Amount of bone recovered after 6 months of reambulation, following 17 weeks of bed rest. Same subjects as in Fig. 23–5. (Data from Leblanc AD, Schneider VS, Evans HJ, et al: Bone mineral loss and recovery after 17 weeks of bed rest. J Bone Miner Res 5:843–850, 1990.)

Tertiary Prevention of Osteoporosis

It is easier to lose bone mass than to regain it after the loss. Specifically, much work is required to regain small amounts of bone mass, especially if the mass is lost due to complete immobility or a sedentary lifestyle. More bone mass is lost during the condition of immobility (due to lack of loading) than in the sedentary state (minimal activity). Walking slows the loss, and high-impact loading can actually increase bone mass (Table 23–1). Clinical conditions producing complete immobility must be addressed with primary preventive measures to minimize bone loss, and secondary and tertiary preventive measures to recover lost bone mineral.

Causative Mechanisms

Mechanical strain, such as that encountered during high-impact loading activities and strength/resistance exercises, increases bone formation (Fig. 23–9). According to Wolf's law, bone remodels itself to adapt to increased loads by altering its mass and distribution of mass.

Osteoporosis occurs when bone resorption exceeds bone formation. The increase in IGF-I mRNA and protein expression is consistent with the model that IGF-I generated by osteoblasts in response to mechanical loading may participate in the induction of bone formation, by its ability to induce proliferation and differentiation of osteoblastic cells in culture.[9]

Prostaglandins are produced very early after the administration of mechanical strain in osteoblastic cells.[9] Also, compounds that induce the production of nitric oxide (NO) increase the rate of new bone formation during mechanical loading.[9] There are multiple isoforms of NO synthase (NOS). Expression of endothelial NOS in osteoblasts and osteocytes has been observed, and been shown to be sufficient to stimulate proliferation of osteoblasts in cell culture. The precise links between these processes, however, remain unclear.

TABLE 23–1. Effects of Physical Activity on Bone Mass	
Physical Activity State	**Amount of Bone Mass Change**
Complete immobility	Very large, no abatement
Sedentary	Minimal losses per day, which accumulate to large losses over decades
30 min walking per day	Rate of loss slowed compared to sedentary, but still yearly losses
Resistance loading, high-impact loading	Actual small gains if done routinely

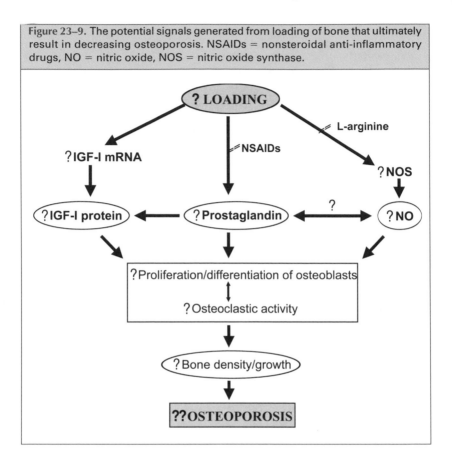

Figure 23–9. The potential signals generated from loading of bone that ultimately result in decreasing osteoporosis. NSAIDs = nonsteroidal anti-inflammatory drugs, NO = nitric oxide, NOS = nitric oxide synthase.

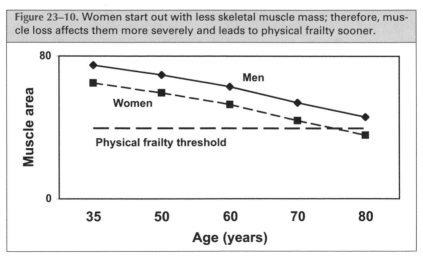

Figure 23–10. Women start out with less skeletal muscle mass; therefore, muscle loss affects them more severely and leads to physical frailty sooner.

Physical Frailty

The occurrence of physical frailty is greater in women than men for the following reasons:

- Women live to an older age than men.
- The magnitude of the peak in skeletal muscle mass at the ages of 30–35 is less in women than men. Since the rate of muscle mass loss with age is similar for both men and women (Fig. 23–10), women will therefore reach the threshold for physical frailty at a much earlier age than men.

Suggested Reading

1. Friedenreich CM, Bryant HE, Courneya KS. Case-control study of lifetime physical activity and breast cancer risk. Am J Epidemiol 154: 336–347, 2001.
2. Thune I, Furberg AS. Physical activity and cancer risk: Dose-response and cancer, all sites and site-specific. Med Sci Sports Exerc 33(6 Suppl):S530–S550, 2001.
3. Lee IM, Rexrode KM, Cook NR, et al. Physical activity and breast cancer risk: The Women's Health Study (United States). Cancer Causes Control 12: 137–145, 2001.
4. McTiernan A. Physical activity and the prevention of breast cancer. Medscape Womens Health 5: E1, 2000.
5. Katz MS. Geriatrics grand rounds: Eve's rib, or a revisionist view of osteoporosis in men. J Gerontol A Biol Sci Med Sci 55:M560–M569, 2000.
6. Leblanc AD, Schneider VS, Evans HJ, et al. Bone mineral loss and recovery after 17 weeks of bed rest. J Bone Miner Res 5:843–850, 1990.
7. Siris ES, Miller PD, Barrett-Connor E, et al. Identification and fracture outcomes of undiagnosed low bone mineral density in postmenopausal women: Results from the National Osteoporosis Risk Assessment. JAMA 286: 2815–2822, 2001.
8. Nelson ME, Fiatarone MA, Morganti CM, et al. Effects of high-intensity strength training on multiple risk factors for osteoporotic fractures. A randomized controlled trial. JAMA 272:1909–1914, 1994.
9. Chow JW. Role of nitric oxide and prostaglandins in the bone formation response to mechanical loading. Exerc Sport Sci Rev 28: 185–188, 2000.
10. Ray NF, Chan JK, Thamer M, Melton LJ III. Medical expenditures for the treatment of osteoporotic fractures in the United States in 1995: Report from the National Osteoporosis Foundation. J Bone Miner Res 12(1):24–35, 1997.

Physiological Regulation of the Human Genome Through Physical Activity

chapter
24

Appropriate Gene Expression

"All that we can do, is to keep steadily in mind that each organic being is striving . . . that each at some period of its life, during some season of the year, during each generation or at intervals, has to struggle for life and to suffer great destruction. When we reflect on this struggle, we may console ourselves with the full belief, that the war on nature is not incessant, that no fear is felt, that death is generally prompt, and that the vigorous, the healthy, and the happy survive and multiply."

~ Charles Darwin, *The Origin of Species*[1]

From Darwin's seminal work, the scientific basis for the concept of how environmental forces directly modify the survival of genes (and thus species) accrued. Our inheritance of genes remains unchanged from the former environment in which physical labor was required to obtain food (hunter-gatherer society), in a pattern of feast or famine. We retain an inextricable connection to our hunter-gatherer genes. This fact must be considered in light of current, comparatively sedentary lifestyles and applied to the understanding of how the environmental-genetic interaction molds our susceptibility to and struggle against the onslaught of modern chronic diseases.

Unequivocal evidence (as presented here in Chapters 12–23) clearly supports the notion that many environmental factors—including physical inactivity—in various combinations are the cause of the majority of chronic health conditions. Indeed, environmental perturbations of genes constitute the causal factors for 58–91% of the three most dominant chronic health conditions (CHCs) afflicting individuals in modern-day America: type 2 diabetes, coronary heart disease, and most site-specific cancers. Thus, the majority of deaths due to CHCs in the U.S. are of environmental origin[9]. Physical inactivity is the second leading cause of death in the U.S., and a contributor to the third leading cause (obesity), and accounts for at least 1 in 10 premature deaths.[9,10]

The intriguing question arises: How does an environmental factor such as physical inactivity trigger the genetic composition of an individual to induce susceptibility to detrimental health conditions, when the genes of humankind have been programmed for maximal preservation by natural selection? Our answer is that environmental factors exert their influence by altering the *expression* of a subpopulation of genes, resulting in a phenotype that passes a threshold of biological significance so that overt clinical symptoms appear—the pathologic state (Fig. 24–1).

Conversely, a certain threshold of physical activity is needed to maintain the proper expression of "physical activity genes." Selection of our genes over 10,000 years ago in our late Paleolithic ancestors established the levels of physical activity required for appropriate gene expression today. Physical activity genes evolved to support the physical labor of survival in hunting and gathering. If this minimal threshold of physical activity is not achieved, then a state of physical activity deficiency ensues, thereby resulting in "pathologic" expression of physical activity

Figure 24–1. Physical inactivity may alter the expression of genes and cause the organism to cross a threshold, beyond which a clinical disorder develops. (Adapted from Booth FW, Chakravarthy MV, Gordon SE, Spangenburg EE: Waging war on physical inactivity: Using modern molecular ammunition against an ancient enemy. J Appl Physiol 93: 3–30, 2002.)

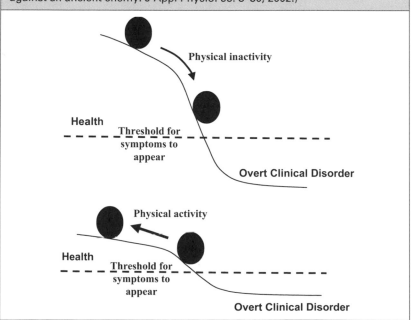

genes that expect, but do not receive enough stimulation. As a result, physical activity genes produce an incorrect amount of proteins that cause overt clinical symptoms of CHCs to appear (Fig. 24–1).

There is both an evolutionary and biologic basis for maintaining a certain threshold of physical activity for the proper functioning and expression of our Paleolithically programmed genes. Modern Homo sapiens are still genetically adapted to a pre-agricultural hunter-gatherer lifestyle because our overall genetic makeup has not changed significantly during the past 10,000 years.[3] Åstrand contends that close to 100% of the biologic existence of humans was adapted to an outdoor existence of hunting and foraging for foods, requiring habitual physical activity.[4] Thus, the portion of the human genome that determines basic anatomy and physiology likely evolved in the physically active hunter-gatherer environment and therefore was largely selected by physical activity.

Consider, too, the influences of the dietary environment. Our hominid ancestors' energy expenditures and caloric intake were higher (206 kJ/kg/day [49 kcal/kg/d]), compared to that of contemporary humans (134 kJ/kg/day [32kcal/kg/d]).[3] Yet our ancestors remained muscular, lean, and physically fit, even though sedentary modern Homo sapiens have a much lower caloric intake than the Late Paleolithic humans. Furthermore, fossil records and epidemiological data from current hunter-gather societies shows that these populations are not developing chronic health conditions such as hypertension, obesity, sarcopenia, hypercholestrolemia, nonocclusive atheromata, and insulin resistance, compared to similarly-aged sedentary populations.[5]

Thus, since the genes are similar in these comparisons, but the amount of physical activity is drastically different, the logical conclusion is that decreased physical activity and decreased caloric expenditure are the paramount etiological factors responsible for the current epidemic of modern chronic diseases. Diet is clearly important, but it is not the sole causal factor. Even though the absolute caloric intake in contemporary humans is lower than in our Late Paleolithic ancestors, it is nevertheless *high* relative to the corresponding decrease in caloric expenditure (compared to the caloric expenditure of our ancestors). The media and much of the scientific community grossly understate the role of physical inactivity. The unfortunate consequence of underemphasizing physical inactivity is an escalation of the epidemics of obesity and type 2 diabetes in our children.

Gerber and Crews[6] assert that those alleles that evolved for function, selective advantage, and survival in the late Paleolithic era are now being exposed to sedentary lifestyles, fat-rich/fiber-poor diets, and an extended lifespan, all of which result in a selective disadvantage with respect to chronic degenerative diseases and longevity (Fig. 24–2).

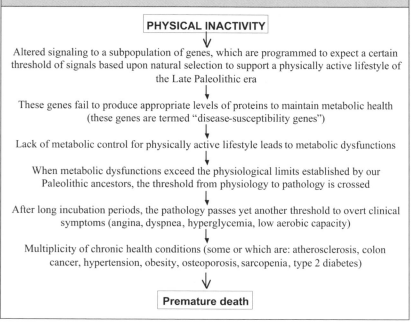

Figure 24–2. Physical activity deficiency produces a dysfunction in physiologic gene expression, such that current U.S. adults have Late Paleolithic hunter-gatherer genes in a sedentary, food-abundant society whose appearance as a culture is less than 200 years old.

PHYSICAL INACTIVITY

↓

Altered signaling to a subpopulation of genes, which are programmed to expect a certain threshold of signals based upon natural selection to support a physically active lifestyle of the Late Paleolithic era

↓

These genes fail to produce appropriate levels of proteins to maintain metabolic health (these genes are termed "disease-susceptibility genes")

↓

Lack of metabolic control for physically active lifestyle leads to metabolic dysfunctions

↓

When metabolic dysfunctions exceed the physiological limits established by our Paleolithic ancestors, the threshold from physiology to pathology is crossed

↓

After long incubation periods, the pathology passes yet another threshold to overt clinical symptoms (angina, dyspnea, hyperglycemia, low aerobic capacity)

↓

Multiplicity of chronic health conditions (some or which are: atherosclerosis, colon cancer, hypertension, obesity, osteoporosis, sarcopenia, type 2 diabetes)

↓

Premature death

Evolutionary Medicine

The notion that the sedentary state does not lead to adverse clinical consequences has no biological basis, and hence is blatantly false. Rather, it is likely that humans have an intrinsic biological requirement for a certain threshold of physical activity. One adverse effect of sedentary lifestyle is a disruption of the normal homeostatic mechanisms programmed for proper metabolic flux needed to maintain health.

Evolutionary medicine asks why the body is designed in a way that makes humans vulnerable to problems like atherosclerosis, a disease whose prevalence only increased in the last 100 years. Many contemporary physical ills are related to incompatibility between lifestyles and genes. For example, in the 1990s, Mexican Pima Indians expended 2100–2520 kJ/d (500–600 more kcal/d in physical activity), had a diet lower in fat and higher in fiber content, weighed 26 kg less, and did not have the diabetes epidemic of their obese Arizonian Pima counterparts.[7] As these two groups only geographically separated 700–1000 years ago, the changes in the prevalence of diabetes between two geographically separate but genetically similar Pima Indian tribes suggest the importance of environmental interactions with the genome.

Genetic Response To the Sedentary Lifestyle

Neel[8] proposed that thrifty genes were incorporated into the human genome because of their selective advantage over the less thrifty ones during earlier phases of human evolution. The selective advantage was increased efficiency of energy storage in periods of food availability, such that the population could survive a future period of famine. Thus, through nearly all of human evolution, physical activity and food procurement were inextricably linked (Fig. 24–3).

We extend Neel's thrifty hypothesis to encompass physical activity. Not only do thrifty genes store food more efficiently in periods of feast, but they conserve blood glucose during periods of apparent energy deficiency (i.e., fasting, physical activity). In sedentary individuals, some thrifty genes express the wrong amounts of proteins and fool the body to think that it is fasting. As a consequence, food stores are misdirected to the adipose, liver, and walls of blood vessels instead of being consumed by skeletal muscles.

Taken together, the macro environment and our sedentary lifestyle affect our cellular environment. Our ancient genes respond to these subcellular changes, resulting in a pathologic over- or under-expression of various gene products and manifesting clinically as modern chronic diseases. It is logical then to presume that primary preventive medicine could reverse

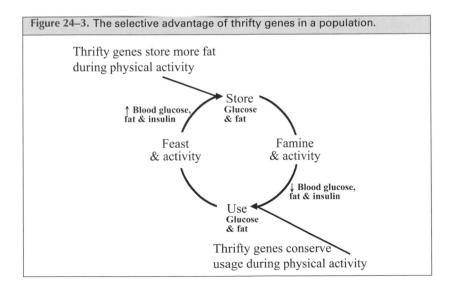

Figure 24–3. The selective advantage of thrifty genes in a population.

Thrifty genes store more fat during physical activity

↑ Blood glucose, fat & insulin

Store Glucose & fat

Feast & activity

Famine & activity

↓ Blood glucose, fat & insulin

Use Glucose & fat

Thrifty genes conserve usage during physical activity

the changes in the cellular environment and diminish or even eliminate chronic health conditions (CHCs) such as obesity and type 2 diabetes.

From a practical point of view, physicians can counsel changes in lifestyle more easily and effectively than they can treat gene sequences in a living human being. Lifestyle changes alone would produce a tremendously positive impact for the 200 million Americans not yet afflicted with a variety of CHCs. Moreover, the 100 million Americans now affected by chronic disorders would, in most instances, benefit from becoming more physically active. Genes were engineered by natural selection to support physical activity to survive. Ironically, underusage of "physical activity genes" results in the physical activity deficiency syndrome, which is non-discriminatory in robbing health from all ages, ethnicities, genders, and socioeconomic groups.

The cost of health care in the U.S. is predicted to double by 2011, and we can't afford that. It also can be contended that it is not humane to treat the patient *after* the overt clinical symptoms appear when primary prevention could have been prescribed. Cure involves not just healing an overt clinical symptom; it also implies *preventing* the clinical symptom. Since sedentary lifestyles produce so much suffering via debilitating CHCs, the progression of which is often relentless, we believe that it the obligation of the healthcare community to practice cure by promoting the primary prevention of chronic diseases with physical activity.

Suggested Reading

1. Darwin C. The origin of species. New York, PF Collier & Son, 1909.
2. Booth FW, Chakravarthy MV, Gordon SE, Spangenburg EE. Waging war on physical inactivity: Using modern molecular ammunition against an ancient enemy. J Appl Physiol 93: 3–30, 2002.
3. Cordain L, Gotshall RW, Eaton SB, Eaton SB III. Physical activity, energy expenditure, and fitness: An evolutionary perspective. Int J Sports Med 19:328–335, 1998.
4. Åstrand PO. JB Wolffe Memorial Lecture: Why exercise? Med Sci Sports Exerc 24: 153–162, 1992.
5. Eaton SB, Strassman BI, Nesse RM, et al. Evolutionary health promotion. Prev Med 34:109–118, 2002.
6. Gerber LM, Crews DE. Evolutionary perspectives on chronic diseases. In Trevathan WR, Smith EO, McKenna JJ (eds): Evolutionary Medicine. New York, Oxford University Press, 1999, pp 443–469.
7. Esparza J, Fox C, Harper IT, et al. Daily energy expenditure in Mexican and U.S. Pima Indians: Low physical activity as a possible cause of obesity. Int J Obes Relat Metab Disord 24:55–59, 2000.
8. Neel JV. Diabetes mellitus: A thrifty genotype rendered detrimental by progress? Am J Hum Gen 14:352–353, 1962.
9. Hahn RA, Teutsch SM, Rothenberg RB, Marks JS. Excess deaths from nine chronic diseases in the United States, 1986. JAMA 264:2654–2659, 1990.
10. Booth FW, Gordon SE, Carlson CJ, Hamilton MT. Waging war on modern chronic diseases: primary prevention through exercise biology. J Appl Physiol 88:774–787, 2000.

Inactivity: A Fat Chance of Being Healthy!

chapter
25

Our major objectives in this book were three-fold:

1. To better define the overwhelming problem at hand. Sedentary lifestyle plays a key role in the drastic burgeoning of many chronic health conditions (CHCs).

2. To trumpet a call to action. We must make physical activity a daily part of our lives and our patients' lives, especially in the segment of the population that is completely sedentary.

3. To outline the biological basis for how physical activity/inactivity affects the pathophysiology of these CHCs.

The salient features of these objectives follow.

Defining the Problem (Chapters 1–5)

According to the U.S. Centers for Disease Control and Prevention, obesity and diabetes are epidemics. Many other chronic diseases are following suit. One in three Americans will be inflicted with some form of CHC. However, the silver lining in the cloud is that many chronic diseases are preventable by simple, cost-effective lifestyle modifications, i.e., engaging in regular moderate physical activity.

Healthcare costs are escalating. The U.S. Department of Health and Human Service's Centers for Medicare and Medicaid predict that healthcare costs will double by 2011, approaching close to 2.8 trillion dollars per year or $9216 per person! We are headed for trouble unless drastic measures are taken to stop this escalation. Eventually, people will not be able to afford proper care. Our book offers a partial solution to this problem: primary prevention of chronic disorders by physical activity.

You may wonder, "Aren't we healthier today due to medical advances?" Yes, we are—in the sense that we are making significant progress in understanding cancer biology, gene therapy, etc. But newer treatments may only benefit the 1–10% of the population who can afford them, and even these individuals will often have to reduce other costs such as savings for retirement, a larger home, a dream trip, or a child's college education. The rest of the population, especially the 44 million currently uninsured Americans, will not benefit from these unaffordable *tertiary* measures. However, *primary* and *secondary* prevention are available to all, and these early approaches must be practiced by the medical community. We plead for increased doctor-patient counseling, community-wide removal of barriers to physical activity, and greater involvement of the federal government in promoting primary prevention of chronic diseases via (a) healthy lifestyle behaviors and (b) regular physical activity.

The Means To Action (Chapters 6–11)

There are now guidelines for physical activity, but they are still evolving. Many of the diseases discussed in this book affect entire populations and are largely a result of lifestyle (high-fat and low-fiber diets, consumption of refined sugar, physical inactivity). Unfortunately, it is the lower socioeconomic groups and the uninsured who are greatly afflicted by these disorders. How are we going to respond to this? Is the U.S. and the rest of the world going to be REactive, instead of PROactive? Being proactive requires prevention of illness before it occurs. Currently, high-risk lifestyles of sedentary days and inappropriate diets are accepted by many because they believe that a pill will be created to replace all of the health benefits of physical activity. This is a major misconception. The widespread health benefits of physical activity on multiple tissues and chronic disorders make it *impossible* to make a single "exercise chemical" for a drug. And even if, by some miracle, an exercise pill were to be made, it would not be affordable for the segment of the population with the highest incidence of obesity, type 2 diabetes, and physical inactivity!

This book is only a beginning to acknowledge the problem of how to primarily prevent CHCs, and this endeavor is an evolving science and art. It is our opinion that healthcare professionals are not trained to address the diverse nature of CHCs to the same degree that they are trained to cure the specific symptoms of acute diseases. This educational imbalance must be fixed.

With the rising cost of prescription medications, soon it will not be practical to indulge in only secondary and tertiary prevention modalities. Healthcare professionals have an obligation to implement preventive programs.

Biological Basis For Chronic Diseases Caused By Physical Inactivity (Chapters 12–23)

One of the most fascinating features of the intricate web of pathways by which physical activity and inactivity modulate genes and, consequently, health is the interconnections. For example, physical stressing of bones, muscles, heart, and brain by physical activity delays/compensates for aging; skeletal muscles' ability to clear blood glucose and fat is lost in 1–2 days by physical inactivity; the entire spectrum of the highly complex metabolic syndrome and whole-body insulin resistance can be initiated by physical inactivity alone. However, note that the purpose of delineating the myriad signaling mechanisms is *not* to find a magic pill or drug. There simply is no substitute for physical activity.

Though we now know that many of the most deadly and debilitating of the CHCs are caused, in part, by physical inactivity/sedentary lifestyle, and that the human body requires physical activity for the proper functioning and expression of its genes, it is a great irony that we still know so little about *how* physical inactivity causes disease and physical activity results in health. It is indeed most unfortunate that there is so little governmental and medical support for research to discern these crucial pathways, if for nothing else other than to further advance the frontiers of our basic knowledge.

We need to establish a solid biological basis for many of the phenomena described in this book. Once there is even greater biological evidence of how physical activity modulates genes and their function and we better understand their complex interactions, perhaps more interest, energies, and monies will be devoted to this unappreciated and under-researched area.

Medical and legal practice demand evidence, but the biochemical and molecular links between physical inactivity and CHCs are still being uncovered. Consider the recent U.S. tobacco debacle. Tobacco companies insisted that there was no data to link cigarette smoke with lung cancer. Once the molecular link was published in research journals, the companies were forced to compensate states for the tobacco-causing diseases, to the tune of hundreds of billions of dollars. Many in the medical field appear to be in a state of denial when it comes to the link between physical inactivity and chronic disease and suffering. Physicians typically do not even ask their patients if they are physically active. Many researchers do not find discovering the molecular basis of disease produced by physical inactivity worthy of time or support, even though they support government funding to determine the molecular basis of cancer, heart disease, diabetes, obesity, etc.—all of which are largely caused by physical inactivity!

We strongly caution that you should *not* underestimate the life-saving potency of physical activity prescriptions for the primary prevention of disease, just because there are no randomized controlled clinical trials with physical inactivity being the only variable (except for the Diabetes Prevention Program clinical trial). Physical activity prescriptions have also proven to be beneficial as a secondary prevention treatment modality. We suggest that the Hippocratic oath's commitment to do no harm includes encouraging, advocating, and prescribing appropriate physical activity as a primary preventive medicine.

What Does the Future Hold?

Information presented in this book unequivocally asserts the crucial role of physical activity in the modern therapeutic arsenal for the fight against chronic diseases. Physical activity is a supremely powerful first-line agent, the "drug-of-choice" so to speak, which is both necessary and sufficient to prevent much of the chronic disease that ails our present-day society. There is simply no other "medicine" that has proven as efficacious as physical activity for the primary prevention of chronic health conditions.

In the years to come, we need to routinely prescribe appropriate physical activity for the primary prevention of chronic disease because it is the right thing to do on *every* conceivable level. It is right for individual physicians, their patients, the healthcare profession, the U.S. economy, and, perhaps most importantly, it is the right thing to do for future generations.

Intensity of Physical Activity

I. Absolute intensity and volume of physical activity

Volume of physical activity/wk =
absolute intensity × duration / day × frequency / wk

Absolute intensity of physical activity can be expressed many ways.

A. Gross caloric expenditure including resting metabolism

Gross kilocalories (kcal) expended per week:
- 140-lb (64-kg) person walking 3 mph will burn 4 kcal/min
- Therefore, 4 kcal/min (absolute intensity) × 30 min/day (duration/ day) × 5 days/wk (frequency/wk) = 600 kcal/wk, which is the total volume of physical activity per week, expressed in kcal.

B. Net caloric expenditure including resting metabolism

For prescribing physical activity for body weight control, only those calories above resting metabolism count toward physical activity–expended calories. Therefore, the caloric expenditure of resting metabolism must be subtracted.
- 140-lb (64-kg) person walking 3 mph will burn 4 kcal/min. However, 1.25 of the 4 kcal/min is for resting metabolism. Thus, net calories expended in physical activity would be: 4 kcal/min–1.25 kcal/min = 2.75 net kcal/min.
- Therefore, 2.75 kcal/min (absolute intensity) × 30 min/day (duration/day) × 5 days/wk (frequency/wk) = 412.5 kcals/wk, which is the total volume of net physical activity per week, expressed in kcal.

291

C. Caloric expenditure expressed as METs

MET-min expresses kcal per week in the units of MET-min, where 1.25 kcals/min = 1 MET (resting metabolic rate)

- 4 kcals/min ÷ 1.25 kcals/min/MET = 3.2 METs
- Therefore, 3.2 METs (absolute intensity) × 30 min/day (duration/day) × 5 days/wk (frequency/wk) = 480 MET-min/wk, which is the total volume of physical activity per week, expressed in MET-min.

MET-hours expresses kcal per week in the units of MET-hr

- Therefore, 480 MET-min/wk ÷ 60 min/hr = 8 MET-hr/wk
- Table 1 illustrates a more practical approach to translating METs into daily activities and physical conditioning.

As mentioned throughout this book, the ability to perform higher METs of work translates to decreased morbidity from disease and a significant reduction in all-cause mortality.

II. Relative intensity of physical activity

There are five ways to express relative intensity of physical activity.

Percentage of maximal oxygen uptake: Percentage of maximal calories burned during the work. Oxygen used to produce ATP for work is an indirect measurement of calories expended by the work.

Percentage of oxygen uptake reserve: Corrects percentage of maximal oxygen uptake by subtracting one MET of oxygen. The strategy is that resting metabolic rate is not added to caloric expenditure to estimate added physical activity.

Percentage of maximal heart rate: Clinical shorthand for percentage of maximal oxygen uptake. Both oxygen uptake and heart rate increase linearly with increasing exercise intensity.

Percentage of heart rate reserve: Corrects percentage of maximal heart rate by subtracting resting heart rate from the exercise heart rate.

Perceived exertion: Patient's subjective rating of relative work intensity.

- **Maximum intensity** declines 1% each year of aging in sedentary individuals (it only declines 0.5% each year in physically active individuals, and decreases 25% after 3 weeks of continuous bed rest in healthy young men).
- **Exercise prescription** must also consider the relative intensity of the work to be prescribed because the relative intensity of walking 3 mph increases with aging. The functional significance is that

Category	Home	Occupational	Recreational	Physical Training
Very light (< 3 METs or < 4 kcal)	Basic ADLs Driving automobile Desk work Cooking	Sitting Standing (store clerk)	Billiards Croquet	Walking (2 mph) Stationary bicycle (very low resistance)
Light 3–4 METs or 4–6 kcal	Raking leaves Painting Scrubbing floors	Light cleaning or carpentry Carrying objects of 15–30 lb	Slow ballroom dancing Golf (cart) Horseback riding Fishing	Walking (3–4 mph) Level bicycle (6–8 mph)
Moderate 4–6 METs or 6–8 kcal	Easy digging in garden Climbing of stairs (slow) Sweeping floor with broom	Shoveling dirt Using heavy power tools Carrying objects of 30–60 lb	Tennis (singles) Golf (walking)	Walking (4.0–4.5 mph) Bicycle (9–10 mph)
Heavy 6–9 METs or 8–10 kcal	Heavy shoveling Climbing of stairs (moderate speed)	Shoveling ditches Manual farm labor Carrying objects of 60–90 lb	Fencing Touch football Swim laps	Jogging (5 mph) Swimming (crawl stroke) Rowing machine Bicycle (12 mph)
Very heavy > 9 METs or > 10 kcal	Shoveling heavy snow Climbing of stairs (fast)	Lumber-jack; Heavy laborer Carrying objects of > 90 lb	Handball Squash Cross-country skiing	Running (> 6 mph) Bicycle (> 13 mph or up hill)

TABLE 1.   MET Values For Daily Activities

Modified from Thompson PD, Ainsworth BE, et al (eds): Exercise and Sports Cardiology. New York, McGraw-Hill, 2001; and Ainsworth BE, Haskell WL, Whilt MC, et al: Compendium of physical activities: An update of activity codes and MET intensities. Med Sci Sports Exerc 32: S498–504, 2000.

the length of exercise time until fatigue is inversely related to the maximal oxygen uptake. For example, individuals running the 100-yard dash exercise have a shorter time until fatigue than if they walked a long distance.

- **Table 2** classifies physical activity intensity, based on physical activity lasting up to 60 minutes.

TABLE 2.   Relative Intensity of Physical Activity Based On the Type of Activity In Various Age Groups

	Type of Activity						
	Endurance						Resistance
	Relative Intensity		Absolute Intensity (METs) in Healthy Adults*				Relative Intensity**
Intensity	Heart rate reserve# (%)	Max heart rate (%)	Young (20–39 yr)	Middle-age (40–64 yr)	Old (65–79 yr)	Very old (80+ yr)	Max voluntary contraction (%)
Very light	< 20	< 35	< 2.4	< 2.0	< 1.6	≤ 1.0	< 30
Light	20–39	35–54	2.4–4.7	2.0–3.9	1.6–3.1	1.1–1.9	30–49
Moderate	40–59	55–69	4.8–7.1	4.0–5.9	3.2–4.7	2.0–2.9	50–69
Hard	60–84	70–89	7.2–10.1	6.0–8.4	4.8–6.7	3.0–4.25	70–84
Very hard	≥ 85	≥ 90	≥ 10.2	≥ 8.5	≥ 6.8	≥ 4.25	≥ 85
Maximal‡	100	100	12.0	10.0	8.0	5.0	100

* Absolute intensity (METs) values are approximate mean values for men. Mean values for women are approximately 1–2 METs lower than those for men.
** Based on 8–12 repetitions for persons under age 50–60 years and 10–15 repetitions for persons aged 50–60 and older.
‡ Maximal values are mean values achieved during maximal exercise by healthy adults.
# Values are similar for percent oxygen uptake reserve.
Data from Fletcher GF et al: Exercise standards. A statement for healthcare professionals from the American Heart Association. Circulation 91(2): 580–615, 1995.

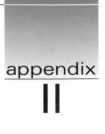

A Sample Physical Activity Prescription Chart

appendix II

Historical information

Exercise history

_____
_____
_____
_____

Barriers to undertaking physical activity

_____
_____
_____
_____

Relevant medical history

_____
_____
_____
_____

Interventions

Methods to overcome barriers

_____
_____
_____

Type of physical activity recommended
☐ resistance
☐ aerobic
☐ flexibility
☐ balance
Duration/volume _____
Frequency _____
Intensity _____
Safety considerations _____
Potential adverse effects _____
Monitoring progress
BP: _____
HR: _____
Ht/Wt/BMI: _____
Waist Circ.: _____
Activity goals: _____
Feedback points/Adherence issues

_____
_____
_____

Referral to multispecialty group
☐ nurse practitioner
☐ exercise physiologist
☐ obesity specialist
☐ cardiologist
☐ endocrinologist
☐ nutritionist
☐ behavior psychologist

Composition of a Low-Calorie Diet

For Overweight/Obese Individuals	
Nutrient	**Recommended Intake**
Total calories	500–1000 kcal/day *reduction* from usual intake
Total fat	≤ 30% of total calories
Saturated fat	8–10% of total calories
Monounsaturated fat	Up to 15% of total calories
Polyunsaturated fat	Up to 10% of total calories
Cholesterol	300 mg/day
Protein	~15% of total calories
Carbohydrates	≥ 55% of total calories
Sodium chloride	2.4 g of Na or ~6 g of NaCl per day
Calcium	1–1.5 g per day
Fiber	20–30 g per day
From http://nhlbi.nih.gov/guidelines/obesity/e_txtbk/index.htm	

HOT TOPICS

Index

Page numbers in **boldface type** indicate complete chapters.